Raising Happy, Healthy, Weight-wise Kids

Raising Happy, Healthy, Weight-wise Kids

Judy Toews and Nicole Parton

With a foreword by Barbara Coloroso

Illustrations by Graham Harrop

KEY PORTER 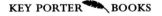 BOOKS

Canadian Cataloguing in Publication Data

Toews, Judy, 1946–
    Raising happy, healthy, weight-wise kids

Includes bibliographical references and index
ISBN: 1-55263-179-6

1. Children – Nutrition. 2. Children – Nutrition – Psychological aspects. I. Parton, Nicole. II. Title.

RJ206.T63 2000   649'.3   C00-931609-4

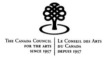

The Canada Council   Le Conseil des Arts
for the Arts   du Canada
since 1957   depuis 1957

The publisher gratefully acknowledges the support of the Canada Council for the Arts and the Ontario Arts Council for its publishing program.

We acknowledge the financial support of the Government of Canada through the Book Publishing Industry Development Program (BPIDP) for our publishing activities.

Key Porter Books Limited
70 The Esplanade
Toronto, Ontario
Canada M5E 1R2

www.keyporter.com

Design: Peter Maher
Electronic formatting: Heidy Lawrance Associates

Printed and bound in Canada

00 01 02 03 04   6 5 4 3 2 1

No one can take away what Nature has given.

Christine de Pizan, c. 1363–1431,
The Book of the City of Ladies,
Persea Books, New York, 1982

Contents

Foreword

For the past thirty years, I have spent a good deal of my time talking about, writing about, and thinking about children. I have three of my own—all grown now—and have spoken to hundreds of thousands of parents in countries all around the world.

I believe that there is something profoundly satisfying about sharing a meal with your children. Eating together, breaking bread together, is one of the oldest and most fundamentally unifying of human experiences. Mealtime rituals vary from culture to culture and family to family. But no matter the culture or family, a child's relationship with food can affect every aspect of his or her life. Weight, whether considered too high or too low, can affect body image; body image can affect self-esteem; and a strong sense of self is one of a child's most important resources when faced with problems, challenges, and temptations.

The development of this strong sense of self is the theme of *Raising Happy, Healthy, Weight-wise Kids.* The authors—Judy Toews and Nicole Parton—believe, as I do, that what we teach our children about choices and decisions related to nourishing their bodies will directly affect the way they feel about themselves and how they interact with the world around them. When our children fall into the trap of thinking that they must look like, act like, or be like a model, sports hero, or celebrity, they are setting themselves up for needless disappointment, and could easily be putting their health at risk.

What can we, as parents, do to help our children avoid falling into such a trap? If you're reading this book, you're already on the right track. In the pages that follow, you'll benefit from the authors' advice and experience. You'll learn how to listen to your body, how to understand what it is telling you about hunger and satisfaction, and how to teach your child to do the same. You'll learn that your feelings about your own body—and the way you express those feelings—do have an impact on your children. You'll learn that your eating, exercise, and relaxation techniques set a very important example, and that a "do as I say, not as I do" attitude will get you nowhere fast.

I know that children carry the lessons they learn at home— from infanthood through the often trying teen years—into adulthood and into the world. *Raising Happy, Healthy, Weight-wise Kids* is a great resource to help you guide your children through the myriad of choices they'll face and the decisions they'll need to make at every age. When your children leave home, they will have the inner resources, the knowledge, and the wisdom to make healthy, responsible, and constructive choices—for themselves and for the next generation that they will create.

—Barbara Coloroso, author
kids are worth it! and
Parenting Through Crisis
June 2000

A Word from the Authors

From Judy:

Many years of experience and countless heartwarming moments—as both a nutritionist and mother—have shaped this book. Almost daily, I advise parents about how and what to feed their children. But nothing has been more challenging or rewarding than bringing up kids of my own. When I was a new mom, I once told an audience that my baby lapped up all the nutritious foods I offered. A voice from the back of the room sang out, "Wait 'til she's two!" Yes, I had a lot to learn about feeding children. Luckily, my daughters Sarah and Erica—now delightful young women—always managed to keep me "real" and make life wonderful.

It's good to be writing about children with my childhood friend Nicole Parton. Nicole's journey to a satisfying weight and sound body image inspired our first book *Never Say Diet!* In it, her personal story is interwoven with my "body sense" principles for healthy living. Once again, Nicole has proved to be inspiring. I don't know whether it was her 25 years as a hard-hitting journalist or her own special brand of wonder that sparked questions such as, "Where does mothers' milk come from and how does it get there?", but the book has clearly benefited.

Life has taught us both that humor can help you get through just about anything, which is why Graham Harrop's marvelous cartoons grace the following pages. Laughter is healthy—that's one of nature's most important lessons.

From Nicole:

Having had three children in the same calendar year (don't ask!), I'll never forget what it was like to be a busy mom. I learned a lot about feeding kids over those first few difficult years, but I also learned what interesting, inquisitive, and complex creatures children are. They deserve our love and respect, and we are privileged to have them as part of our lives.

In editing this book, I've learned a great deal more about feeding kids—body and soul—from my longtime friend Judy Toews. I look forward to the day that I can use my newfound wisdom as I cradle my first grandchild. We hope you enjoy reading—and living—this book. It was written by and for people who love children.

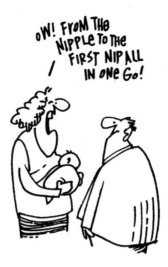

From the Nipple to the First Nip

Sometimes it seems as if the whole world is on a diet. It's never been more fashionable to be thin, yet many of us—even children—are heavier than ever. Today's kids face two weight-related issues: Childhood obesity has doubled in the last 20 years, and millions of kids who *are* at healthy weights feel dissatisfied with their bodies.

Six-year-old girls want to be ultra-slim. Ten-year-old boys long for lean, muscular bodies. Even three-year-olds complain about feeling "fat" in their snowsuits! Youngsters of all sizes and ages are eager to look like models, movie stars, or sports heroes—a desire that can lead to eating disorders, smoking, drug use, and disillusionment.

Weight concerns can make life miserable for kids. A child who becomes preoccupied with physical appearance is a child who no longer hears that brave inner voice that says, "I can do it!"

Many parents worry that their kids are too big or too small, or that they eat too much or too little. Those who've struggled with their own weight anxiously watch their children for signs that history is repeating itself. One mom I spoke with at a kindergarten clinic anguished over what she realized was a paradox: "She's bigger than her friends! I'm afraid she'll have a weight problem like I do. And yet ... she's so picky, I worry she's not eating enough!"

I reassured her that normal, healthy kids come in all sizes, which means some are bigger and some are smaller than other kids the same age. Likewise, normal, healthy children have a range of appetites. Although "picky eating" is typical at some developmental stages, it can become entrenched if no one helps a child learn to like a variety of healthy foods.

I hope this book will reassure you, too. As a parent, I understand why people fret about their child's eating habits and body size. As a nutritionist, I know parents often worry too much. It's a challenge to identify real weight and feeding problems without jumping to the conclusion that every larger- or smaller-than-average child *has* a problem. It's another challenge to address weight-related issues without stigmatizing a child as being too big or too small. It's a fine balance—but it's not as difficult as it may seem.

From infancy, our bodies signal their need for the basics of balanced living—food, movement, rest, relaxation, love. Paying attention to these inner signals can give you a sense of how much food, exercise, sleep, and relaxation you need. If you're out of step with your body's "inner wisdom," it's hard to send the children in your life the spoken and unspoken messages that promote healthy living.

Amidst the chaos of day-to-day life, it's easy to lose touch with your built-in knowledge of what's right and wrong for your body. By presenting practical insights based on Nature's lessons, this book will show you how to tune in to your bodily needs—and how to help your child listen to her body, too. A child who is "in tune" with her body is more likely to have a healthy weight and positive outlook, whatever her size or shape. In simple terms, she'll be "weight-wise." (Because weight issues affect both girls and boys, this book alternates "she" and "he," chapter by chapter.)

This book will also help you create the right circumstances and opportunities for healthy living, both inside and outside your home. That means providing healthy food at regular intervals and allowing kids to respond to their bodies' needs by deciding whether to eat, and how much. It means encouraging kids to keep active, without going to hazardous extremes. It means helping them find the middle ground between rusting out and stressing out. Perhaps most important of all, it means helping kids accept and respect themselves—while accepting and respecting others, too.

How can Nature's lessons for healthy living help your child achieve a natural weight and positive body image? Nourishing food and pleasurable activity are two pieces of the healthy-weight puzzle. Ease of body, mind, and soul is the third. Think of them as the "3 E's": Eating well, Exercising for fun, and Easing relaxation into everyday life.

Don't underestimate the importance of that third "E." Stress can make you settle for low-quality food. It can make you eat too much, too fast—or not at all. It can make you too tired, fearful, or apathetic to plunge into activities. It can make a toddler throw a tantrum in the grocery store, or a teenager drink and drive. Today, more than ever, our kids need to learn how to relax and be easy within their own bodies and minds.

We live in a confusing, contradictory world of super-size servings and stingy diets. Along with television programs featuring super-slim characters, kids watch ads for fries, burgers, pizza, soft drinks, candy, and beer. TV exposes them to 400 food commercials a week—and countless role models. Bombarded with media messages about how to look and what to eat, many kids tune out those all-important inner messages that tell them when they're hungry and when they've had enough.

From the nipple to the first nip, food represents comfort and love. But as a child grows, food can also become a pastime, a babysitter, a friend—or an enemy. Weight and body-image problems are endemic among our children: Some kids are running on empty, while others aren't running at all. Today's kids spend more hours in front of televisions, video games, and computers than they do in school. Inactivity allows bodies to weaken and minds to grow sluggish; it also contributes to the increasing incidence of childhood weight problems.

We can blame our crazy mixed-up world for all of these problems, but hand-wringing won't help! While we can't change the world overnight, we *can* do something about our own attitudes, and the way we influence kids. This book will alert you to your attitudes about food, exercise, stress, weight, and body image—whether you're a parent, teacher, childcare worker, doctor, coach, celebrity, hero, or several of the above!

When adults adjust their attitudes about body weight and do their best to encourage balanced living, children benefit. It's been said that it takes a village to raise a child. It always has. Relatives, friends, neighbors, teachers, and peers play a part. So do the pervasive influences of television and other mass media, including music videos, movies, and magazines. Today's kids feel as if they know their heroes—and they want to be just like them. The magazine photo may be airbrushed, the model may have an eating disorder, the athlete may take steroids, but the image is beautiful and the admirer wants to emulate it. Back in the "village," we have our work cut out for us—unless we can convince celebrities and others to promote diversity and size acceptance.

Where to begin? It's easy to feel overwhelmed by the sheer volume of parenting information out there. But it's worth remembering that parenting is a skill we learn "on the job." We all want to get it "right." I always encourage parents to listen to their heads *and* hearts—in fact, to their entire bodies!

It was more than 50 years ago that Dr. Benjamin Spock initiated a parenting revolution with the simple words: "Trust yourself. You know more than you think." As a parent, you do often know what's best. You may learn a great deal from others, and even more from your own experience. You also have "gut feelings," or know some things in your "bones." Long before there were parenting experts, there were parents attuned to their "inner wisdom."

Implicit in Spock's advice to "trust yourself" was the idea of trusting your child as well. We soon learn we can't control everything that affects our children. We want the best for them but can't always be there to guide them. In today's "village," youngsters transfer some of their loyalty from caregivers to peers at a very early age. Cooperative play in childcare centers, play schools, and kindergartens fosters attachment to the group—and the group has its own ideas, influences, and enticements, both good and bad.

Nature's lessons for living can help you and your child sort out the differences between the good, not-so-good, and just plain awful influences on your relationship with food. They can also help you show your child how to live a balanced life. As your child grows, she'll learn to make her own choices—and you'll learn to let her. While children don't need us to make all their decisions, they *do* need our guidance and support. As a parent, you simply can't do it all—and you'll do your child a huge disservice if you try. She needs practice to become a good decision-maker on her own!

Don't wait for the "right time" to explore Nature's lessons. That time is now. It's never too soon to think about health-related issues—prevention can begin even before a child is conceived. It's also never too late for parents and kids to become fitter, stronger, healthier, and wiser. The human body is amazingly resilient. Did you hear about the former couch potato who became a personal trainer? Or the 70-year-old who started running in her 50s and now competes in marathons? How about the five-year-old picky eater who later became a nutritionist? (Not to mention any names!)

In Part I: A Growing Concern, you'll learn about the wide-ranging influences on your child's weight and body image. In Part II: "E"-sy Growing, you'll learn to help your child form weight-wise habits at each developmental stage by following the 3 E's: healthy eating, exercise, and ease.

"Nature always wins!" reads the newspaper headline about a hurricane. Yes, Nature demands our respect. Just as treetops sway in a storm, Nature bends—but won't be ignored! Using Nature's lessons to raise a child is a bit like gardening. It's messy and labor-intensive, but the right amount of food, water, sunshine, and love virtually assure a strong root system.

I can't think of anything more satisfying than watching a child bloom. Like flowers, our children can reach for the sky, but we also know it's important that they remain firmly grounded. We dream they'll become healthy, happy, and wise—the best they can possibly be! This book is dedicated to all the children in your life and ours. May they touch the stars while staying rooted in a healthy, nurturing world!

PART I

A Growing Concern

1
Eating for a Living

Nature is a brilliant architect. Our bodies
were designed to signal their need for food.

Eating is one of the most intimate things we do. We take food into our bodies—thousands of pounds over a lifetime—and it becomes part of us. From birth to 18 years, your child will eat something like 33,000 meals and snacks. This chapter explores the reasons kids eat the way they do.

It's easy to overlook the full significance of food. At times, it's simply fuel—there when we need it, at home or at stops along the way. In our hurried lives, some of us eat not only on automatic pilot, but even on overdrive.

Food is much more than something that fills us up. As you feed your baby, comfort, love, gratification, and survival are forever intertwined. Food helps to forge a strong, enduring link between you and your child. The cozy snuggle as you feed your infant. The toddler's look of wonder when you present the birthday cake. The call from a college student who misses your cooking. These are memories parents cherish. But life has its ups and downs. Your child may also invite himself to the neighbors' house because they're having packaged macaroni and cheese and you're cooking fish. At times, he'll stare into a well-stocked refrigerator and claim there's nothing to eat. I've been there!

Food affects every aspect of your child's life: his growth, development, behavior, intelligence, immune system, and sense of well-being. His eating experiences in early childhood may give rise to food and weight issues in adolescence. Chronic dieting, eating disorders, poor self-image, and "out of control" behavior can some-times be traced right back to the cradle. But this book isn't about blaming parents—or anyone else. It's about understanding how problems develop, so they can be prevented or corrected. It's also about celebrating the joy of "breaking bread" with the kids in your life.

Sharing the Power

Feeding children is an awesome responsibility, but it's one we share with our kids. Surprised? Let me explain what I mean. As a parent, it's your responsibility to provide healthy foods for your child. *But deciding whether to eat—and how much—is your child's responsibility, right from infancy.* Staying clear on these separate roles is an essential part of raising a child with a healthy weight and positive body image. The idea of shared responsibility is one I'll come back to again and again. Developed by child-nutrition guru Ellyn Satter, it's a cornerstone of this book.

Well-meaning parents often attempt to take on both jobs: They not only provide the food, they try to get their kids to eat it, too! Parents who can't cajole their kids to eat sometimes call me at their wits' end. I tell them to stop coaxing. Nature's blueprint calls for children to eat when they're hungry and stop when they're satisfied.

With practice, a new parent can learn to interpret an infant's signals for hunger and satisfaction. Following the rule of shared responsibility also helps older babies and toddlers feel secure about eating. It lets you share the joy of discovery with a primary-grade child, and it teaches a budding preteen to trust his body. It prepares a full-fledged teenager to mesh his yearning for independence with good sense.

Sharing responsibility with your kids is good for you, too. You really don't have to do it all! Pressuring yourself to make your child eat is both frustrating and futile. No one can *make* a child eat—at least not without a battle that spoils the meal. When you do your part and let your child do his, it's a win-win situation.

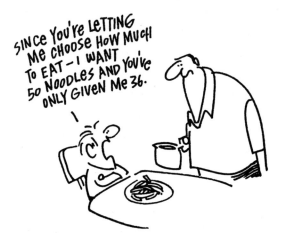

Body Wisdom

We are all born with body wisdom that helps regulate our eating. At least 40 signals run between the gut and brain to indicate when we need nourishment. Babies read those signals loud and clear. After all, they're not distracted by work, worried about their waistlines, or swayed by commercials. They can't tell time, so they certainly don't know when it's customary to eat!

From childhood to the teen years and beyond, people who "listen to their bodies" seem to know just how much to eat without depending on outside cues. Even when there's chocolate cake left on the plate, they'll often put down their forks saying, "That was good! I've had enough." They seem to be able to eat whatever they want, whenever they want, without gaining extra weight. Forget food scales and measuring cups—paying attention to your body is by far and away the best method for deciding how much to eat.

Eating is not just a basic instinct. It involves learning, right from the start. Since it usually takes between one and three hours to digest and assimilate food, we don't really know how satisfying something will be until some time after eating. When we repeatedly eat a certain food, we unconsciously "learn" just how filling it is. This allows us to anticipate how much the food will fill us up, and adjust the amount we eat.

This process begins very early in life. Babies as young as six weeks can adjust the amount they drink according to their meal's "energy density"—its concentration of calories. Studies show that by six months of age, with no prompting from their moms, breast-fed babies may start to eat their largest meal at night, before going to sleep. Up until that time, babies tend to eat more in the morning, particularly if they've gone several hours without food. The switch may be a response to subtle changes in their mothers' milk. How else would a baby (even a very smart one!) know he needs extra food to get him through the night? Changes in the composition of breast milk in the evening may send a signal to babies to increase the amount they take. Bottle-fed babies don't do this, because formula doesn't change from one meal to the next. (Never tamper with the concentration of infant formula; always mix *exactly* according to package directions.)

You can help your child respect his appetite and respond to the energy density of his meals at each stage of his development. Start by paying attention to the signals your infant sends you about his hunger or satisfaction. Long before your little one learns to talk, he'll have an amazing capacity to communicate. He'll raise his arms in the air, and you'll know he wants to be picked up. In one recent study, babies not old enough to speak learned basic sign language! Babies are also telling us something when they clamp their mouths shut and turn their faces away at mealtime. The message is clear: He's had enough! Don't "make an airplane" with the spoon or coax the poor dear to have just one more bite "for Spot." (If you do, don't be surprised when he starts slipping parts of his dinner to the dog!) Remember the principle of shared responsibility? You offer food; your child decides whether and how much to eat. If you forget, your child's behavior will soon remind you!

As your child gets older, you can talk to him about how hungry or satisfied he feels. If you push your child to eat when he's not hungry, reward him for finishing food, or punish him for leaving food, you'll teach him to ignore his body signals. It's also wrong to withhold food or otherwise discourage a hungry child from satisfying his appetite. When that happens, a child begins to focus on getting food wherever and whenever he can—it's a natural impulse for survival. A child who's not allowed to respond to his body's signals must rely entirely on outside cues to tell him when and how much to eat. Studies show that the more authoritarian the parent, the poorer a child's inner regulation of food intake.

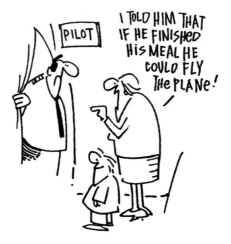

Banning Bribery at Your House

"Eat your carrots, Mark, and you can have a cookie." "If you sit on your potty like a good girl, Kirsten, Mommy will give you two Smarties."

If you bribe your kids to do what you want them to do, what do they learn? Mark may choke down his carrots to get a cookie, but he's not learning to like carrots. Kirsten may perform on the potty to get some candy, but she's not learning that it feels good to respond to her body's urges. Instead, Mark and Kirsten are learning how to "earn" rewards. One mom told me her child tried to spin out his potty time so he could get more candy!

There's an obvious downside to making food a reward for good behavior, but parenting educator Barbara Coloroso advises against giving kids any kind of prizes for doing what should come naturally. We give toddlers stars and stickers for "being good" and by the time they're teenagers they want to know what they'll get for doing a chore or making the grade at school. I overheard a new high-school graduate say, "My parents can pay my college tuition—they're the ones who want me to go."

Give your kids treats and support them in any way you can—just because you love them. But don't teach them that life is about getting prizes for doing the right thing.

Like many adults, you may be a little rusty at listening to *your* body. After years of responding to outside cues, you may have forgotten how to recognize real hunger. And the signals to *stop* eating are even subtler! If you depend on diets and other outside influences to tell you how much to eat, you probably end up alternating between eating too little and too much—neither of which is very satisfying. Diet plans simply can't offer the kind of precision our bodies need to balance the calories we take in with the calories we use up.

Studies show that parents who have difficulty regulating their own eating often have kids with the same problem. Chronic dieters—whose eating problems may be rooted in their own childhood experiences—may inadvertently set the stage for their children to become dieters, too.

There's plenty of evidence that young children know when they're hungry and can gauge how much they need to eat. But do they have a natural ability to choose specific foods to meet their needs? Pioneering studies conducted by U.S. pediatrician Clara Davis in the 1920s and 1930s are often cited as evidence that infants know instinctively what to eat—even though Davis herself didn't draw that conclusion.

Davis offered her subjects a variety of fresh, unseasoned, unprocessed foods and let them choose whatever they wanted. All selected a combination of foods in amounts that helped them grow normally. What would have happened if she'd offered them cookies, candy, chips, and ice cream? It's safe to assume that, given the chance, Davis' subjects would have gone straight for the sweet and salty treats, because infants show a preference for those flavors. In fact, Davis did report that vegetables were her subjects' least favorite foods. No studies have been able to show that children instinctively know *what* they need to eat. They may be good at gauging *how much* they need, but kids need their parents and other caregivers to provide a healthy variety of foods at regular intervals throughout the day.

I Taste, Therefore I Eat

Most babies enjoy sweet foods and reject sour and bitter substances right from birth. Could this preference be one of our built-in survival skills? Mother's milk is sweet, while poisons are often sour or bitter.

A preference for salty foods begins at around four months. Given the human body's need for sodium, a taste for salt makes sense—although too much isn't healthy. Unfortunately, food manufacturers often add salt in copious amounts, hoping to enhance the products' appeal. Parents do the same thing when they salt their babies' food.

Although many kids would like to, your child can't live exclusively on sweet and salty foods. Acceptance of other flavors seems to come down to experience—some of it very early in life. Babies are exposed to different flavors even before they take their first mouthful of food. While Junior is still floating inside the womb, he's swallowing amniotic fluid—the liquid that makes up his environment. Since this fluid is flavored by the food Mom eats, Junior may be getting a head start on developing his food preferences.

It's not surprising that breastfed babies are more open to trying new foods than those accustomed to swallowing the same formula every day. Because it's flavored by the food a mother eats, breast milk doesn't taste the same at every meal. Mom may be eating lots of different things with an interesting variety of flavors. Breast milk varies in other ways as well. During feeding, the fat content of breast milk changes, with the rich milk at the end of the feeding providing an important source of essential fatty acids and energy. For that reason, a mom should let her baby completely empty one breast before switching sides. As a child's nutritional needs change over time, the nutrient composition of mother's milk also changes.

The more flavors your child experiences, the better. Children who get used to a varied diet are much more likely to try new foods, creating an ever-expanding base from which they can meet their nutritional needs. The three most important characteristics of a healthy diet? Variety, variety, variety!

Ah, but there *is* a catch! Helping kids learn to like a variety of foods can be tricky, especially when they show a natural inclination to reject unfamiliar foods. This "neophobia," or fear of something new, offers yet more evidence of an instinct for survival. When your baby splutters with the first yummy taste of mashed carrots, be ready for it. Don't be dismayed when your toddler shoves away a lovely dinner and shouts: *"No!"* Both are perfectly normal behaviors. Kids may also become increasingly leery of new foods as they get older. The innocent babe may swallow anything soft you put on a spoon, while the savvy two-year-old keeps a sharp look out for the unfamiliar.

Working with Your Baby's Instincts

A baby who's learned to grab and hold will instinctively pop whatever he finds into his mouth. A crawling baby can find dust-encrusted bits of food and lost toy parts that are almost invisible to the adult eye! As you rush about trying to make your child's world safe, consider this phase another part of Nature's plan. Your baby will perfect his hand-to-mouth action around the time he starts to need a wide variety of foods. This is what educators call a "teachable moment." If he likes to put things into his mouth, he's ready to learn to eat (watch for guidelines in Chapter 5). Your baby's natural tendency to chew on things also makes teething easier. A hard, cold object—such as a teething ring chilled in the freezer—can ease the pain.

Introducing new foods takes plenty of patience. Most taste preferences are developed through repeated exposure. You may have to offer a child a new food 15 or 20 times over several weeks or months before he accepts it. Don't give up after one or two tries. It's easy to end up catering to children, preparing separate meals on a daily basis. That's a disservice to kids and parents alike.

Generally, children have more taste buds than their parents, making them extra sensitive to strong flavors (maybe that's why one cooked cabbage will serve six adults or 297 preschoolers!). Some kids inherit a tendency to be "super-tasters." Their extra taste buds make strong vegetables taste even stronger. This may explain why finicky eating seems to run in families. Expect most kids to take their time learning to eat vegetables—and don't worry if your "super-taster" declines when you pass the broccoli. One night he may discover it tastes great stir-fried—especially if a friend or older sibling tucks right in.

Taste preferences are also linked to cultures and traditions. While today's worldwide "youth culture" has made soft drinks and hamburgers universal favorites, many food preferences come from years of tradition. Mischievous Nepalese kids are more likely to hide something hot and spicy in their school desks than a chocolate bar or bag of candies. Green peppers are a traditional favorite with children from India (although I once knew an Indian family whose five-year-old didn't want to eat anything but McDonald's hamburgers!).

Don't be surprised if you run up against the occasional food jag. All week long, Baby loves peas. The next week, he won't touch them! Because kids are naturally wary of new foods, they sometimes prefer to fill up on one thing, especially if it's a favorite. The less hungry they are, the more likely they'll shun less-preferred foods. Food jags end when a child tires of the food he's been favoring—an understandable result of sensory overload.

Some kids are more accepting of new foods than others. As preschoolers, my nephews would eat any kind of shellfish, cheerfully counting the accumulation of empty shells. My kids—eyeing clams and mussels with suspicion—would reach for the noodles. We all know of lucky parents who can brag that their child eats everything. Then there are the desperate ones who call me saying, "Help! My child won't eat *anything*. He's living on air!"

Rest assured there's not one documented case of a child living on air! The fussiest kids always eat something. Although it's not unusual to find toddlers who favor liquid diets and preschoolers who restrict themselves to a handful of foods, it's never as hopeless as it seems! The baby who clamps his mouth shut when he sees a spoon *can* learn to take solid food. With a little guidance, the toddler who's fallen into the habit of sipping juice all day can become an educated eater. The school-aged child who refuses to eat a packed lunch can be shown there's life beyond hot dogs. The teenager who decides to eat vegetarian can learn to balance his meals. In the pages to come, you'll find as much emphasis on *how* to help kids eat healthfully, as on *what* foods to offer them.

Let the Good Times Roll!

Besides having a natural inclination to enjoy sweets, children especially like foods they associate with good times—and dislike foods they link with bad experiences. It's no coincidence that fast-food ads beckon us with promises of good times and fun!

Take cake, for example. Not only does it taste nice and sweet, but it's served at parties. No one has to coax kids to eat it. It's pretty and tasty and everyone enjoys it. Sometimes, cake is even a reward for being "good," or for eating something else first.

Compare that with the way a family presents everyday foods. There's no excitement, no singing, no candles, no pretty decorations. Just Mom and Dad trying to coerce Junior to eat something that's "good for him." Sometimes they even argue about whether he should have to eat it!

Pity the poor brussels sprout. Not a party food. Rarely a reward for good behavior. You have to eat it before you can have dessert. It tastes strong—especially to "super-tasters." It's not sweet or salty—no match for a cookie or a crunchy chip. Even Mom or Dad may dislike it!

A team of U.S. researchers offered two groups of children a new drink, each in a different way. Kids in one group were rewarded for downing it. Those in the other group simply sampled it several times. The kids who were rewarded after drinking the beverage were less inclined to like it! In fact, pressuring *or* rewarding children to eat or drink something can make them *dislike* the food or drink.

Just before Easter one year, I presented a nutrition workshop to a group of primary teachers. One—who had planned to serve the usual chocolate treats at her class party—saw an opportunity too good to miss. She gave the children cardboard and scissors and showed them how to make cute Easter Bunny ears. As they sat in a circle wearing their new ears, she read them a story about rabbits. Then they played some rabbit games. Their snack? Carrot and celery sticks. You should have seen those bunnies munch their "rabbit" food! Nobody asked for candy.

Now, I don't believe that candy and cake should be "forbidden foods" (one reason being my fondness for chocolate!). Those primary-school students probably had some candy at home, and that's fine. But their teacher didn't need to reinforce their appreciation of sweets. Because she understood how children develop food preferences, she decided to support healthy food choices by making vegetables fun.

You can do the same thing. In Chapter 5, we'll explore how you can help kids of all ages learn to enjoy a wide variety of healthy foods, without making foods high in sugar, fat, and salt seem even more desirable than they already are. In the meantime, remember nutritionist Ellyn Satter's "golden rule" of shared responsibility:

Parents and other caregivers are responsible for offering a variety of nutritious foods, in appropriate places, in a pleasant manner, at regular times throughout the day. Children are responsible for deciding whether to eat, and how much to eat at each meal and snack.

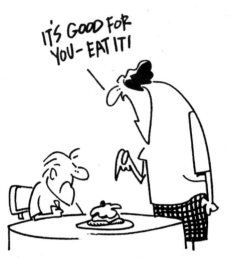

ANOTHER WAY To MAKE JUNK FooDS UNDESIRABLE To CHILDReN

Because You Asked Why Kids Eat the Way They Do

Q: Breast-fed babies are supposed to know how much to eat, but I think my daughter may be eating too much. Everyone says she's a big baby. Should I limit her time on each breast?

A: *Trust your baby to eat until she knows she's had enough, letting her empty the first breast before moving her to the second. Let her be the one to decide when to stop nursing—she'll feel frustrated if you take her off the breast before she's finished. Your little one needs to learn that she can depend on her body to let her know when to* *start and stop eating. Your baby's size is partly determined by genetics. For your peace of mind, talk to your doctor or public health nurse about your daughter's growth pattern.*

Q: Dinner is a battle of wills. Nick, our six-year-old, loathes green beans. It's a fight each time we have them. My husband makes him sit at the table until every bean gets eaten—no matter how long it takes or how much he cries and gags. This doesn't seem right, but we can't think of a way out.

A: *Instead of learning to like green beans, Nick is learning to dislike mealtime. Seek a truce and enlist your husband's support. Like many well-meaning parents, he's trying to get your son to eat. But that's Nick's responsibility. When you're serving green beans, ask Nick if he'd like some. If he declines, don't discuss it further, but continue to offer them—and anything else you prepare—once, at the beginning of the meal. Allow Nick to help himself to food at the table and don't coax him to eat. He'll be more cooperative about trying new things if he doesn't feel pressured or afraid of being punished. Dinner will be more pleasant for all of you!*

Q: I was always taught to clean my plate and reminded about the world's starving kids. If I let my kids decide how much to eat, they'll leave too much food on their plates. How can I avoid waste?

A: *"Cleaning your plate" can mean overriding your appetite and losing touch with your body's ability to regulate eating. It won't help the world's starving kids, either! Minimize waste by letting your children serve themselves at the table, taking the amount they expect to eat. Suggest they take a small portion first, then have more if they're still hungry. If a child's "eyes are bigger than his stomach," let him put his leftover dinner in the fridge to eat later as a bedtime* snack, but don't make him have it for breakfast! Save untouched leftovers (promptly pop them in the fridge or freezer at the end of the meal). If they're not suitable for tomorrow's lunch, freeze them for the next time you make soup.

Q: My kids spend their entire allowances on junk food. Should I let them get their "fix," or encourage them to make better choices?

A: *If the "junk" food isn't taking the place of healthy meals, take a low-key approach. It's what your kids eat overall that really matters. It's great for them to learn to handle money and perfectly normal for them to enjoy newly found consumer power. Consider encouraging them to save half their allowances for something special. Offering to match the amount they save—especially if it's for a big-ticket item—may motivate them to redirect some of their funds to more worthwhile purchases.*

Q: By the time I get home from work, my teens have already snacked until they're full and have lost interest in dinner. Any ideas?

A: *Eating dinner together is a wonderful way for you and your teenagers to stay in touch. Dinners are also likely to be more varied and nutritious than snacks. Without hassling them, get your teens involved in the meal. Ask for their input in planning dinner, and let them decide how to cut back on snacks. Ask them how (not if!) they'd like to help—to set the table, make a salad, chop the veggies, prepare a marinade, turn on the barbecue, make a simple dessert. And when they do help, let them do things their way. If they want candles, go for it! Listen to their favorite music during the meal (you get to control the volume!). Have fun!*

2
Family Matters

*Nature creates relationships, inspiring in parents
a deep desire to respond to children's needs.*

I once watched a boy about six dawdle over breakfast at a restaurant, while his mother read a magazine. Every few minutes she looked up and told him to eat. Finally, she slammed down her magazine, hacked his pancake into chunks, and stuffed a forkful into his mouth. Poor kid. His mom thought she had to get food into her son—whether he wanted it or not. Her actions showed him he needed to eat to please *her*, rather than satisfy his own needs.

Another time, I overheard a pair of solicitous parents read an entire menu to a preschooler. She couldn't begin to decide, so they reread several sections. I had to restrain myself from peeking over the booth and suggesting they offer the bewildered child a choice of two or three selections. These parents may have been more respectful than the mom who force-fed her child, but they weren't any more responsible. They expected their three-year-old to make *all* the decisions about eating.

A child's experiences around eating, exercise, and ease begin at home. Regardless of outside influences, *your* attitudes about food, fitness, and self-esteem will profoundly affect those of your child.

It's a changing world. The huge influx of women into the paid workforce over the past 40 years has redefined parenting. Family time often means a ride to childcare, or a drive-through meal on the way to a soccer game. As a parent today, you're charting new ground: You can't simply bring up your child the same way your parents raised theirs. That means you'll have to make some conscious choices. This chapter will focus on the role that family dynamics plays in raising healthy, happy kids.

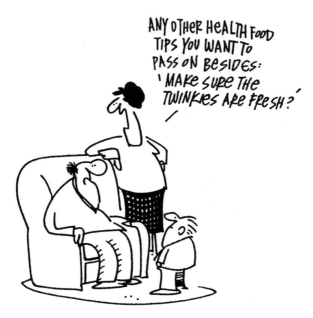

The Mother Load

When I was a young mother, I used to say that working part-time gave me the best of both worlds: time to spend with two delightful daughters, and an opportunity to have an interesting, challenging career. Occasionally, I had the worst of both worlds. Time crunches at work. Not enough energy to do all the things stay-at-home moms did. When my husband took the girls camping for a few days, I accomplished so much I wondered if being married with children was all that stood between me and a Nobel prize!

There's no such thing as a part-time mother. Once a woman has a baby, that child is part of her life, 24 hours a day, seven days a week. Whether a mom stays at home or plunges into the workforce, she's destined to juggle a multitude of tasks. It's convenient that the female nervous system seems to adapt so well to diverse demands—except that it's easy to take on too much.

Perhaps you're the sort of woman who drops off the videos and runs through the car wash while in labor and heading for the hospital. It's great to be versatile, but "supermomitis" can lead to burnout. If you want to be healthy and strong, prioritize—and ask your partner and kids to share the load. That's "share" the load, not "help" you out! Trying to be a supermom is self-defeating, and it doesn't set a healthy example for your kids. Both boys and girls learn a lot about what it means to be a woman by watching and listening to their mothers and other role models. Take some time for yourself—at least 30 minutes a day—and show your children that real women pay attention to their own needs, too!

The way you express your feelings about your body also sends a powerful message to the kids in your life. Too many children hear their mothers, aunts, neighbors, and teachers fretting about their weight and appearance. Young moms are often surprised when I advise them not to criticize their bodies in front of their kids. Mothers of boys sometimes think I'm not talking to them! After a moment, the idea sinks in. None of us wants girls *or* boys to think that women's bodies should conform to the dictates of fashion. Most of all, we don't want our children to feel there's something wrong with *their* bodies. I like the beauty secrets attributed to the late Audrey Hepburn: For attractive lips, speak words of kindness. For lovely eyes, seek out the good in people. For a pleasing figure, share your food with the hungry. For beautiful hair, let a child run her fingers through it once a day.

Millennium Man

Fathers need brand-new job descriptions. These days, dads are often active in the care and feeding of their children—but they're not always certain what to do. Take the example of the dad who brought his four-year-old daughter into a convenience store. "What would you like for dinner?" he asked. "I don't *want* dinner!" was the heated reply. "I hate dinner! I don't want it!" Father and daughter eventually bought potato chips and beef jerky—and went off without dinner. Dad no doubt had mixed feelings about those food choices, but would a traditional authoritarian approach have helped? Probably not.

Social scientists claim that men often feel torn between their desire to be caring and gentle, and what they see as a responsibility to discipline their kids. Women also experience these conflicting pressures, but we're more accustomed to talking to each other and asking for advice.

Steering a Middle Course

One of my colleagues—a public health nurse—spoke to me about a new mother determined to "do everything right" when it came to feeding her child. Unfortunately, the baby wasn't going along with the plan. "I wish the mom wouldn't try so hard," said my coworker. "Things go smoother when parents are more laid back."

Why is that? It hardly seems fair. We put them to bed at the "right" time in the "right" way—but they might not sleep. We offer them the "right" foods in the "right" way—but they might not eat. If they do sleep and eat the way we want them to, we feel successful. If they don't, we think we must be doing something wrong. Steering a middle course means not getting too attached to either outcome. Your child may cooperate; she may not. Don't let your ego get in the way.

Steering a middle course means guiding a child, without demanding that things go your way.

Just like mothers, fathers need support systems—especially if they're single parents. Balancing work and family commitments isn't easy. Raising kids affects parents' jobs, and single parents, in particular, feel the crunch. They may have to take time off to care for sick kids, or give up a promotion that would require relocation or longer hours. This can be especially trying when self-worth is tied to one's career, as it often is. Asking for help—advice, moral support, assistance with chores—is hard for a person who considers the need for support to be a sign of weakness.

The good news is that men seem to be spending more time with their kids. A recent Australian study found that fathers spent an average of 10 hours a week alone with their children in 1998, compared to one hour a week in 1983. The results point to an important shift in priorities. In the more recent study, fewer fathers ranked their role as breadwinner first; more found the most important thing was being accessible to their kids, as well as guiding and teaching them.

I once knew a pediatrician who was a devoted father. For many years he ate broccoli, although he never managed to acquire a taste for it. When his youngest child became an adult, he gave it up—telling his surprised wife and children that he had eaten broccoli only to set a good example!

Here's some advice for dads: You don't have to eat something you don't like for two decades to be a good father! Just be aware that what you say and do—as well as what you *don't* say and do—can influence your child's eating habits. If you refuse to eat something, or seem suspicious of new foods, don't expect your child to be an eager eater. Unfortunately, kids aren't always keen about foods their parents enjoy. But a positive attitude about whatever's served will help set a pattern for pleasant family mealtimes.

Your attitudes about body shape and size are just as important as your feelings about food. Daughters are particularly vulnerable to comments about body weight—whether in general, or specific to them. Boys are also becoming increasingly body conscious. I guarantee that your comments about people's bodies, whether disparaging or complimentary, will not go unnoticed in your home.

United We Stand!

There's really no need to get caught up in the differences between mothers and fathers. It's much more important to emphasize the need for cooperation between them. Not surprisingly, studies show that the stronger the relationship between husband and wife, the better the communication between them, and the greater the husband's involvement in the household. Your child will benefit if you and your partner take some time to nurture your own relationship. (Some parents today are *too* child-focused. When the kids grow up—which they do in the blink of an eye—parents who've directed all their attention to their children may no longer have much in common with each other.)

It's harder for parents to cooperate about eating when they don't live together. Much harder. But believe me, it's worth the effort. It's essential to your child's health and happiness that both parents agree on what foods to offer, and work together to encourage healthy eating. It doesn't matter if Dad has better cooking facilities or Mom has limited culinary skills. It doesn't matter if one has more time or more money than the other. It's essential to agree on a basic routine that's suitable to both households. Kids can handle minor variations in that arrangement, but it's hard to deal with power struggles between Mom and Dad.

Even before a child is born, a woman is encouraged to eat right and take care of herself. When I was pregnant, my husband used to say he did *his* part cheerfully! Joking aside, partners need to cooperate about the food and substances both consume. A pregnant woman who has her partner's support and encouragement will find it much easier to follow a healthy lifestyle. From conception

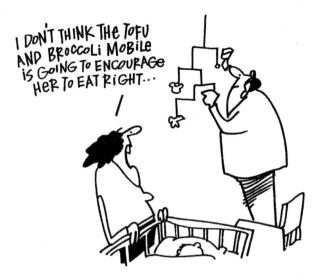

I DON'T THINK THE TOFU AND BROCCOLI MOBILE IS GOING TO ENCOURAGE HER TO EAT RIGHT...

on, both parents-to-be share the responsibility of creating the right environment for bringing up a healthy child. A single parent who lacks a partner's support should seek it elsewhere—from friends, family, or within the community. As I've previously said, it "takes a village" to raise a child, every step of the way.

Family lifestyle is important—but it isn't the only issue. Without blaming or judging, talk to your partner about attitudes related to body weight and size. During pregnancy, discuss how you both feel about your weight gain—and your expectations for getting your shape back after the baby is born.

You may find it reassuring to discuss your feelings about body size and body image at prenatal classes. At the very least, be sure to discuss it at home. These issues will come up again and again, and they can affect both your self-esteem and your relationship with your partner. The "house attitude" about body size and shape will also send a key message to your child as she grows and develops.

Try to be as frank as possible about your opinions. Does someone's size or shape influence how you feel about that person? Do your standards of what's acceptable differ for boys and girls, men and women? Have you ever told a "fat" joke or scoffed at some-one for being skinny and weak? What words do you use to describe people of various sizes? Are the words positive, neutral, or negative? There's no need to blame; we're all products of our culture. This is a time for consciousness-raising and cooperation.

If either you or your partner has ever worried about weight, one or both of you may be anxious about the possibility of your child inheriting a tendency to be over- or underweight. Read this book together. Remember: Although genetics does play a role in body weight, your family lifestyle is at least as important.

Self-esteem vs. Sylph-esteem

The more you trust your parenting instincts, the more confident you'll become. Confidence is a powerful tool that enables us to make the most out of life. It's also something you can pass on to your children!

True confidence comes from within. As you learn to trust your own judgment, you develop self-esteem. "Sylph"-esteem—the sense of worth that comes from external qualities such as the way you look—is the opposite of self-esteem. Because it's based on some-thing transient, sylph-esteem doesn't tend to build your confidence. Bodies change, fashions change, and so do life circumstances.

Poor self-esteem lies behind some of the most devastating problems kids face. Eating disorders and drug abuse wreak havoc on too many young lives. In my experience, kids who feel worthy tend to keep themselves on a path to balanced living. They may be curious about diets, drugs, and alcohol. They may be inclined to test the limits and learn from their experiences. But kids with high self-esteem have a solid foundation. They believe in themselves, and they're able to see and respect the worth of others.

Children's self-esteem starts to develop when they're babes in arms, and someone notices and responds to their need for affection, food, rest, and play. Reinforce your child's confidence every chance you get—confidence to know when to eat and when to stop; confidence to play hard and work hard; confidence to reach for the stars!

Sure, the world beats us down sometimes. We walk out of the house feeling great and someone sneers at our shoes. We study really hard, and still fail the test. That's what makes parents and other significant adults so important to kids. In the boxing ring of life, you're the trainer in the corner, the one with the towel and the water and the words of encouragement.

Helping Your Child Cope with Bullying

Teasing and bullying are a daily reality for many kids. Sadly, those who are teased may begin to pick on others. As a parent, you can teach your child strategies for coping.

Most children don't like to think of themselves as bullies. Simply learning that pushing, name-calling, and excluding are forms of bullying may prompt some kids to stop mistreating their classmates. If your child feels she's being taunted or victimized, encourage her to avoid bullies and play where there's good supervision. It's also important for children to ask for help if they don't feel safe. That means knowing the difference between tattling and talking about what's happening to protect themselves, or to protect someone else. It's tattling to say: "Brian's eating candy in class." It's not tattling to say: "Callie's calling me names," or "Jon tripped Alex and laughed when he fell down."

Kids can learn to be assertive, although it's best to back off in a dangerous situation. Help them practice looking someone straight in the eye and saying, clearly and firmly: "Carter,

stop teasing!" Ask your child's school counselor about training to combat bullying in your area. Excellent programs
are now available in many schools and communities.

If your child is larger or smaller than average, she'll need
plenty of support and encouragement from her family. She'll
need to know that people who tease her or call her names are
ignorant, whether or not they mean to hurt her feelings. She'll
need to hear lots of compliments—on her strength or gentle-
ness, her zany sense of humor or quiet sensitivity, her generosity,
her kindness. Helping her to become aware of all her special
attributes will build her confidence and enhance her life in
countless ways.

Older kids and teens are particularly vulnerable to others'
ideas about body size. As your child grows up, your steady support
will continue to be important. Think of your son's or daughter's
confidence as a little flame. Your job is to gently fan that flame,
taking care not to let anything or anyone blow it out.

Because You Asked about Family Lifestyle

Q: I want to get pregnant, but I'm concerned that if I put on too
much weight, I won't be able to take it off. I saw a photo of a
model in her third trimester, and she barely had a bump!

A: *During pregnancy, nourishing your baby will be your most important responsibility. The model in that photo runs the risk of having
a low-birth-weight baby with potential health problems. Your doctor
or prenatal instructor will help you monitor your weight gain so
you won't feel out of control. If you're anxious about weight gain,
be sure to say so. You'll find your health professional's guidance*

reassuring. After your baby's birth, exercise (brisk walks with baby!) and breastfeeding will help you return to your pre-pregnancy shape. Breastfeeding puts extra body fat into milk production, and stimulates the uterus to quickly return to its usual size.

Q: By the time I leave work and pick my kids up from daycare, I'm beat. I try to cook several vegetables every night, but it's not easy. Sometimes I end up getting takeout—but it's hard to avoid high-fat food. Please help.

A: *Keep those meals simple, Mom. Make your priority unwinding and enjoying being with your kids at dinnertime. I applaud your determination to give them several vegetables, but go easy on yourself. Cook vegetables together in the same pot, toss them in with the noodles, or serve them raw. Mix and match several kinds of frozen veggies—they're nutritious and don't require washing and chopping (for maximum nutrition and minimum cost, stick with the kind without sauces). Let the kids help with dinner so your time together starts as soon as you get home (see Chapter 5 for age-specific suggestions). Don't feel guilty about buying a little convenience. Pick up a deli chicken, bake potatoes in the microwave, and add an instant salad made from packaged greens. Whatever the meal, light a candle and celebrate the pleasure of eating together!*

Q: I'm divorced. When the kids visit their dad, it's fast food all the way. They think this is cool, but I'm simmering!

A: *Chill out, m'dear! Enlist your ex's cooperation in making some compromises so there isn't such a contrast between meals with each parent. The kids can still eat well if Dad suggests milk instead of a soft drink, a protein food such as meat or cheese as part of the main course, and a piece of fruit instead of a sugary, high-fat dessert. Keeping to a pattern of regular mealtimes is important, too, since growing bodies need a steady source of nutrients and energy.*

Once in a while, maybe Dad would consider having a "regular"
meal, and you could treat the kids to dinner out.

Q: Our supermarket offers pint-size "customer in training" carts
for kids. It's fun to shop with my daughter, except when she
tries to fill her cart with junk food. Any suggestions?

A: *Avoid in-store arguments by deciding before you leave home what*
foods your daughter may put in her cart. Make a list for each of
you (if she can't read yet, let her draw hers). Allow her to choose
between two similar foods, such as Cheerios or Shredded Wheat,
smooth or crunchy peanut butter, red apples or green ones. If she
takes lunch to preschool or daycare, let her select some of the things
she'll pack. Before going down the aisles, teach her to steer her
cart around the perimeter of the store—where you'll find most of the
basics. You may want to cap the trip by letting her choose a healthy
treat such as a pack of sugarless gum or a natural fruit bar.

Q: My son Joshua could use a boost to his self-esteem. He's a
quiet, shy 10-year-old who's heavier than most kids his age.

A: *Never miss a chance to tell Joshua what a great guy he is—to*
let him know you love and appreciate him just for being him.
Compliment him when he listens to his body, eating when he's
hungry, drinking when he's thirsty, playing and taking breaks to
relax. For an added boost, help him feel successful with a new
hobby or activity, perhaps one that includes his friends. Encourage
him with sincere compliments such as, "I think it's great the way
you can really stick with it when you're building a model. That
takes patience," or "It was neat the way you talked to Uncle Andrew
about your collection. You're really good at explaining things." Take
every opportunity to help Joshua feel good about all his personal
qualities and skills. When he makes mistakes, help him see that
everybody else does, too. That's how we learn!

3
Telekiddies

*Nature glories in diversity. Like the
birds and flowers, human beings display a
boundless variety of sizes, shapes, and colors.*

Families matter—but no family is an island. Hundreds of people play a part in your child's life. Thousands more influence him through mass media. This chapter examines outside influences—television, magazines, peer pressure, school life—and their potential effects on your child's weight and body image.

North American children spend more time watching TV than doing anything else except sleeping. This daily exposure can affect eating habits, activity levels, and self-esteem. The better we understand how TV exerts its influence, the better equipped we are to counter negative messages and support a healthy childhood.

Predictably, kids who watch a lot of TV are also attracted to other sedentary-yet-entertaining pastimes, such as sitting at the computer. Everyone from tots to teens is exploring cyberspace. There's even a Web site for babies (or maybe their parents) that displays a series of simple patterns meant to calm a fussy infant held up to the screen. According to a recent survey conducted by Time and CNN, 40 percent of American teens have logged onto the Internet, with the number growing daily. The interactive capacity of computers is both exciting and frightening. Joey may be researching his latest science assignment, but he's just a few keystrokes away from pornography and hate literature. And then there are video games. The same poll says one in three boys may be addicted to them. Is computer use more stimulating than watching TV? Perhaps. But the seat of the pants remains firmly applied to the seat of the chair—and moving fingers don't burn many calories.

Television, computers, and other outside influences aren't necessarily harmful. In fact, they can enrich your child's life, provided you set some limits and help him to maintain balance among competing interests.

Prime Time?

Pediatricians' groups in Canada and the U.S. warn that children under two are better off without television. But in some parts of the western world, babies as young as four months watch almost an hour of TV daily. Moreover, a recent study showed a third of parents of two-and-a-half-year-olds are convinced their children can distinguish between reality and fantasy on TV, as well as differentiating between ads and content.

Are they right? It's hard to say. Still, it's remarkable how quickly children learn what's real and what's imaginary on television. Experts say kids unconsciously pick up subtle clues that help them make the distinction. Ask children what's real on TV and they'll say, "The news." One of the reasons news reports seem credible is that the reporter or anchor looks straight at the camera, making "eye contact" with the viewer.

Talk shows dominate daytime TV. Do kids consider them "real" because the host looks straight at them? Talk show hosts wield extraordinary influence, although they attract their following in a rather ordinary way—by sharing personal thoughts and experiences. Icons Oprah Winfrey and Rosie O'Donnell—bright, talented women and role models for millions—frequently focus on their personal weight-loss struggles. Imagine the impact on kids when the much-admired Oprah or Rosie—already successful, popular, wealthy, and powerful—places so much importance on getting thin.

Even though kids know soaps and sitcoms aren't real, they're still swayed by the antics of their favorite characters. Unfortunately, television doesn't provide many lessons in healthy living. Actors are more likely to sip coffee or guzzle beer than eat a balanced meal. And you don't often see someone playing a sport, washing a car, or walking a dog. These days, TV often portrays stressful situations. Good-bye, Beaver Cleaver. Hello, Bart Simpson!

What are kids doing as they soak up TV's messages? In many cases, absolutely nothing. Watching television is such a passive diversion that a viewer's metabolism can drop below its usual resting rate (can you spell "z-o-m-b-i-e"?). That means a child may burn fewer calories watching TV than reading a book, putting together a puzzle, or even sleeping! Of course, the more time kids spend watching TV, the less time they spend walking, running, jumping, skipping, and climbing. It seems as if television "deprograms" their natural inclination to move about. Sitting around perpetuates sitting around. All of the action is on the screen.

Television undermines weight-friendly living in still another way: It exposes kids to hours and hours of commercials, whetting their appetites for high-calorie, low-nutrient foods. Food ads affect what kids eat, how they eat, and when they eat. Commercials prompt kids to eat while they're watching TV, whether or not they're hungry. And a child tuned in to a TV program isn't tuned in to the inner signals that regulate his eating.

One study of children's Saturday-morning TV viewing found children exposed to an average of one food ad every five minutes. Not surprisingly, none was for vegetables! The most commonly advertised items included candy, soft drinks, chocolate products, whipped toppings, cakes, cookies, and pastries. Advertisers turn the basic food guides upside down, encouraging kids to choose the least nutritious foods the most often.

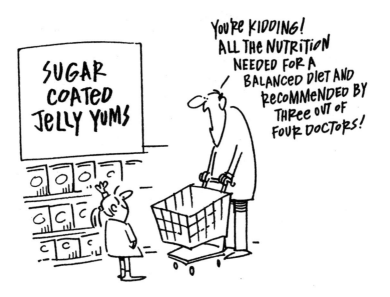

It's not surprising that the more kids watch TV, the less healthy their overall diet becomes. Advertising works. Studies show that the foods most frequently advertised are the ones children request most often. The more kids watch TV each week, the more advertised foods they request—and the more their parents buy.

Kids also influence their parents' purchases of everything from movie rentals to vacations. We have a long tradition of caving in to "pester power!" More than 20 years ago, I read a study claiming 80 percent of parents bought the breakfast cereals favored by their preschoolers. Today, children also have more money in their pockets than ever before. Some teens spend $500 a month on CDs, clothes, and snacks—that's more "disposable income" than many adults enjoy!

The advertising industry in the U.S.—which in the mid-1990s spent $130 billion—has been called the "most powerful educational force in America." And kids constitute one of the strongest consumer groups in the western world.

Fashion Rules!

Ever get the impression that only women with long legs and men with broad shoulders become doctors, lawyers, and police officers? Actors, models, entertainers, and popular sports figures often "fit the mold." How easy it is for young people to get the impression that everyone in the world is more beautiful and glamorous than they are! The media offers us a marked lack of diversity in body types.

Celebrities seem to be less "real" these days. Over the past 20 years, beauty pageant contestants and *Playboy* magazine center-folds have become progressively thinner. The typical Miss America contestant now weighs 13 to 19 percent less than the average North American woman, in many cases meeting the clinical weight criteria for anorexia nervosa. Plastic surgery enables legions of underfed, narrow-hipped bodies to sport large breasts. First there was Barbie—now, there are people who *look* like Barbie. Well, almost. If Barbie were life-size, she'd be seven feet tall with measurements of 38-18-33!

Today, it's more difficult than ever for kids to come to terms with their developing bodies. Even before puberty, they're thrust into a highly sexualized, competitive, frenetic world in which tape measures and scales gauge a person's worth. The "standard" is almost impossible to achieve.

U.S. healthy-weight advocate Frances Berg says girls and women now consider weights in the lowest five percent of the healthy-weight range to be "ideal." That excludes the other 95 percent. Years ago, models' bodies were meant to be unobtrusive "coat hangers"—racks for the clothes they displayed. Today, models are personalities in their own right. We know their names. They have fan clubs. Girls identify with them, and want to look like them.

Reading fashion magazines should be fun, but a psychology study in the mid-1990s found that 70 percent of readers felt dissatisfied with their own bodies after five minutes of reading. Meanwhile, a Boston study revealed that more than two-thirds of girls in grades five through 12 felt they should "measure up" to the images in magazines. Although fewer than a third could be considered "overweight," nearly half the girls surveyed said magazine photos made them want to lose weight.

Reality check: Many magazine images are simply unreal. Everything from starvation to plastic surgery, drugs, and even masking tape is used to shape models' bodies for that picture-perfect look. Airbrushing and other photographic and computer manipulations ensure flawless complexions and cellulite-free thighs. Exposing kids to unrealistic, unhealthy images sets them up for disappointment and even despair. The more a child yearns for "perfection," the harder life becomes.

Adults know that kids are much more than the sum of their physical features. It's heartbreaking to watch a confident, assertive grade-school child become an unhappy, insecure teenager. Dr. Mary Pipher, author of *Raising Ophelia*, believes that girls stop thinking about who they are and what they want when they enter puberty. Instead, they start thinking about how to please others and attract boys. Intelligent teenage girls know there's something wrong with this picture. As one 16-year-old told me, "I feel like a hypocrite. I know it's crazy to get sucked in by media stereotypes, but I care a lot about how I look."

Girls too often feel split into what Frances Berg calls their true and false selves. They can be authentic and honest, or they can be loved and admired. Boys receive mixed messages, too. Desirable men are masculine and aggressive, but society stipulates that men treat women as equals. An obsession with appearance takes both girls' and boys' attention away from how they feel on the *inside*—happy or sad, energetic or tired, challenged or bored—and

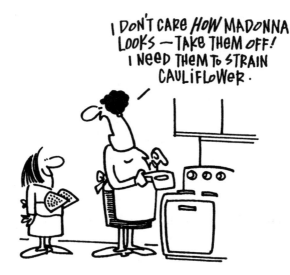

redirects it to how they look on the *outside*. Looking good becomes more important than being relaxed and comfortable, or cutting loose and having fun. Feelings become something to suppress. Kids become competitive with each other instead of supportive, cooperative, and compassionate—qualities that build effective social groups and communities. Ironic, isn't it? While teenaged girls want to be slim and pretty, they often envy and dislike girls who fit that image. The pervasive media influences that turn kids into super-model wanna-bes are at the very root of peer pressure.

Friendly Competition

Our family spent two years in Kuala Lumpur, Malaysia, where the students at our children's school came from more than 100 countries. On that school's "International Day," everyone wore their native dress. At noon, students thronged the cafeteria in sarongs, kimonos, Nehru jackets, saris, and kilts while their mothers served foods such as Thai noodles, sushi, curries, and shortbread. After school, the same kids dressed in T-shirts and jeans to drink sodas and listen to Sheryl Crow. An "all-American" scene!

"Youth culture" is a new phenomenon fueled by worldwide access to western fashion, music, and fast food. In the most remote hill-tribe villages of northern Thailand, boom boxes broadcast rap music to entire communities. The products and messages also reach adults, but it's the teenagers who are most eager to embrace the symbols of North American life portrayed in movies, TV programs, and music videos. It seems as if youths have stronger ties to young people living thousands of miles away than they have to adults from their own culture.

In her controversial book, *The Nurture Assumption*, Judith Rich Harris claims that children influence one another considerably more than their parents influence them. This will not be a revelation to any parent of a teenager! In fact, most of us can remember the force of peer influences back when *we* were teens. Harris contends that parents have very little power to shape their children's behavior. She believes that what children learn at home matters much less than what they learn from others. In effect, Harris reduces the power of parents to suppliers of genetic material: If your kids inherit your traits, they may turn out to be just like you; if your children are adopted, their personalities will more greatly resemble those of their biological parents. You can't shape a child's character—you can only treat him decently and hope for the best.

Harris' premise has been debated in offices, boardrooms, schools, and kitchens. Her book has sparked an outflow of testimonials that either credit or blame parents for the successes and failures of their children. What do you think? If I agreed entirely with Judith Rich Harris, I'd have to trim my advice to two words: Good luck! Happily, there's plenty of solid evidence to indicate that parents can and do make a difference.

Whether or not you can shape your child's character, you still have an opportunity—and a responsibility—to influence the course of his life. Sensitive parents learn early to respond to their children's personalities and quirks. Giving kids the freedom to make choices within reasonable bounds allows them to develop practical skills, regardless of their character traits. Being a parent is more than being a gene bank. What you say and do—and the emotional support you provide—counts. Peers are powerful, but so are you! As U.S. parenting educator Barbara Coloroso says, if you teach your kids to think for themselves, they're not likely to blindly follow the crowd.

What is it about the age in which we live that makes outside influences seem more pervasive than in the past? It may be the way media influences are compounded when everyone watches the same TV programs, admires the same celebrities, absorbs the same commercial messages, and wants the same stuff. That children want to be like other children isn't new. Infants have always found other small people fascinating. Preschoolers have always placed a high value on the friendship, opinions, and approval of their peers. If you want to persuade a four-year-old to try a new food, wait until he's with his playmates. Kids recognize their peers early in life, and will do whatever they can to boost their sense of belonging.

School Cool

As a microcosm of society, schools provide both opportunities and barriers to healthy living. Unfortunately, size prejudice thrives at school. To ensure acceptance, students of all shapes preoccupy themselves with attempts to get—or stay—thin. The fear of being rejected is realistic. Rejection can take the form of subtle looks, snide remarks, or outright harassment. Even some well-meaning teachers tell "sizist" jokes and many more make self-deprecating remarks. Hatred of body fat is one of the last remaining forms of prejudice that's socially acceptable.

Discrimination on the basis of body shape can be devastating for larger-than-average kids. But they're not the only victims. Size prejudice hurts *everyone*. When anyone is put down for being "fat," everyone is afraid to gain weight. Not only does this fear of fat keep kids preoccupied with appearances, it perpetuates unhealthy, unpleasant, degrading diets. What a waste of human potential!

Schools can offer health programs directed at preventing dysfunctional eating, inactivity, and size prejudice, but it's essential that staff be qualified to teach them. That requires up-to-date training by experts in weight management and eating disorders. Programs that perpetuate myths about dieting—or inadvertently show kids how to engage in disordered eating—are counterproductive. Knowledgeable teachers can integrate healthy weight principles with lessons about nutrition, fitness, and sexuality. It takes sensitivity and skill to raise the collective consciousness of the group without making anyone feel self-conscious.

It's important to stay clear on the difference between *teaching* preventive programs and *treating* weight and body-image problems. Teachers can learn the signs and symptoms of eating disorders, but it takes an expert to make a diagnosis and provide treatment. A well-meaning teacher can do a child more harm than good by overstepping the limits of his training and experience.

Schools can promote healthy living in several ways. Breakfast clubs, snack programs, and school lunches help fuel bodies and brains for active learning. But schools that sell lots of high-fat, high-sugar foods contribute to erratic eating and inappropriate snacking. Growing bodies also need daily physical activity. Positive experiences in gym class can lead to a lifetime of fitness; negative experiences can bench kids for years. The ultimate way to support healthy kids is for schools to promote size diversity and show as little tolerance for size bias as for any other antisocial behavior.

Staying Grounded

Most parents do their best to help kids grow up "real," despite the siren call of outside influences. Of course, it's not just kids who succumb to eating more and exercising less, while wanting to be slim and fit. It happens to adults, too. As families, we can turn the situation around.

It's easy to feel overwhelmed by media influences, but parents and teachers can sift through the positive and negative messages and help kids do the same. Maintain the attitude that one size *does not* fit all! Seek a balance between family values and external pressures. Don't try to go it alone: Ask for cooperation from other family members, as well as from teachers and friends. Studies show families that make communication a priority are most likely to have kids with healthy weights. Listen to kids. Share your thoughts with them. The dinner table is a good place to do it. Talk about media influences and about what your kids and others are watching. Let them reflect on it. That reflection can make watching TV more meaningful.

Countering Negative Body Stereotypes

We were seated in a crowded waiting room when my three-year-old suddenly blurted, "Mommy! See that lady?" As I looked up to see a large woman enter the room, Sarah continued: "She has nice long hair just like Mary's." I was relieved that my daughter hadn't remarked on the woman's size. But then, why would she have?

If you treat people of all sizes with equal respect, you can expect your children to do the same. Body size becomes a nonissue. This is an important step toward ending size discrimination. Don't attribute positive qualities to people just because they happen to be slim ("She's a real little dynamo!") or negative qualities to those who happen to be larger than average ("He's a big slob!"). Too often, people incorrectly assume that someone who's thin is self-directed and fit—and someone who's heavy is undisciplined and unhealthy. Studies show that these biases are reflected in some companies' hiring practices and some colleges' admissions! Don't make negative references to your body or anyone else's—including your child's.

Shift your attention from weight toward health and well-being. How we live is more important than what we weigh. *We all* can eat well, live actively, and feel good about ourselves—regardless of body size.

If you've grown accustomed to watching television while eating, ask for everyone's cooperation to turn off the set for 30 minutes so that you can talk instead. Look for ways to focus attention on the real people in your family instead of the characters on TV. If the house seems too quiet and dull without the usual din, play some music. Sometimes TV is simply background noise. Does it stay on even when no one's paying attention? Decide which programs are worth watching—and turn off the set between shows.

Do you know what your child is watching? Provide guidelines for the amount of time he can spend in front of the TV, and for the types of programs that are suitable. What's appropriate for your child will depend on his age and the amount of time he needs for homework and play or activity. Help younger children understand the difference between make-believe and reality on TV. Ask children under eight what "real" means. Encourage kids of all ages to discuss what they see and hear, but don't feel you have to have all the answers. No one does.

Help your child critique advertisements, including food commercials. Let him know that many of the healthy foods you have at home don't need to be advertised—everybody already knows how good they are! Give your child some guidelines on the kinds of foods you're willing to buy, in terms of both nutrient value and cost. You may have to remind him that it's your *responsibility* to ensure he has access to healthy foods.

Supervise your child's Internet use, pointing out material he should avoid. If he communicates with strangers on the Net, make sure he knows how to protect his privacy.

Visit your child's school regularly. Parents often spend more time in elementary schools than in high schools, perhaps because younger kids tend to welcome their visits more than teenagers do. (The first grader loves to have Mom help out at Sports Day. The 10th grader hopes she won't volunteer to chaperone the school dance!) Schools have a huge impact on kids' lives, and children benefit when moms and dads get involved. What kinds of food are available at school? Do what you can to support the availability of healthy choices. I've never heard of a school selling cigarettes—but some sell more soft drinks, chips, and candy than "real" food.

Parents have a positive influence on their children's lives when they respond to kids in ways that are supportive, rather than manipulative. This doesn't mean placing a child on a pedestal and sacrificing your needs to his every whim. It means being clear on the differences between adult and child roles. Remember that you don't need to play both parts. Offer your child healthy food, but don't pressure him to eat. Provide opportunities to be active without forcing him to participate. Coach him on the sidelines, but resist jumping in and taking over. And don't forget to let your child know how *he* can support *you*, too.

If life is a balancing act, then parenting requires the finesse of an Olympic-caliber gymnast. Be *responsive*, but don't feel you should be *responsible* for every aspect of their lives. If your kids propel themselves headfirst into junk culture, the situation calls for balance between your need to protect them and their need for independence. It all comes back to that golden rule of shared responsibility: *Parents set the boundaries within which kids are free to explore.* British Columbia nutritionist Cathy Richards puts it this way: Imagine a house with no fence, perched on the side of a cliff. A yard without boundaries could be a dangerous place for a kid to play. But if the yard is enclosed by a high fence built close to the house, a child could feel stifled, angry, and bored. The best parental boundaries are symbolized by a large yard with a fence the child can see over, and a gate that's sometimes open.

Because You Asked about Outside Influences

Q: Bradley, our five-year-old, always asks for cereals he sees advertised on TV. I buy them because he's a finicky eater and at least he gets his milk that way. (He doesn't like drinking it in a glass.) I let him fix the cereal himself on Saturday mornings. Am I giving him too much control?

A: *Two positive things are happening here: Bradley is gaining some independence by getting his own breakfast on Saturdays, and—as you've said—he's taking milk with his cereal. When you shop, check the labels on cereal boxes and offer Bradley a choice of two or three lower-sugar products. Does your little cereal fan skimp on other healthy foods such as fruits and veggies? Let Bradley have cereal for breakfast and perhaps for a bedtime snack. At other meal and snack times, offer a variety of different foods, including milk products such as cheese and yogurt.*

Q: Our 10-year-old daughter Amanda eats dinner in front of the TV, then goes upstairs to do homework. I eat later when my husband gets home. I enjoy unwinding and reading the paper while Amanda has her meal, but I realize we're having fewer real conversations and she and her dad hardly see each other.

A: *Tell Amanda you'd like to spend more quality time with her. If your husband can make it home by 7 p.m., plan a family meal. Suggest a nourishing after-school snack to tide Amanda over, as well as a head start on homework before her dad gets home. Let her see the show she used to watch at her previous mealtime, so she won't feel she's being punished. If Dad can't make it home by 7, let Amanda eat earlier but sit at the table with her, enjoying a salad or cup of tea ahead of the meal you'll share with your husband. On weekends, make plans for family meals.*

Q: My son is moving next term from an elementary school with an excellent hot lunch program to a junior high that sells a lot of junk food. The principal says kids my son's age need to learn to make choices, and if the school doesn't sell pop and candy, the kids will only buy them at a nearby store. I'm worried my son will find the junk food irresistible. What can a parent do in a situation like this?

A: *Enlist the support of other parents or the school's parent organization to see if students, teachers, and parents might work together to consider some changes. Your local public health nurse or nutritionist may also be willing to play a role. Be sure the students get involved, or the idea probably won't fly. Meanwhile, make it easy for your son to make healthy choices by letting him pack a lunch from a selection of wholesome foods he enjoys. Keep the issue in perspective. If you make too big a deal about school food, your son may not want to tell you what he eats outside your home.*

Q: Our teenage son lives on the computer. When he's not doing homework, he's surfing the Net. He's an intellectual kid who makes good use of his brain, but he doesn't get much exercise. He hates physical education class and refuses to come to the gym with me. Help!

A: *You're wise to encourage your son to become more active. Let him know that his mind will be even sharper if he takes some breaks to revitalize his body. Help him generate a list of activities he might enjoy: cycling to school, walking the dog, learning to play squash, working out at home, swimming. Maybe he could use the Internet to research different options. Suggest he set up a schedule on the computer to keep track of his activities. Perhaps he can help you log your trips to the gym, too. Together, find ways to reward yourselves for sticking with your exercise plans.*

Q: My 15-year-old niece Laura is obsessed with clothes. She used to enjoy challenging novels, but now she reads nothing but fashion magazines. The models are skinny—and the clothes outrageously expensive. How can I get her to "see the light"?

A: *Why not show a little interest in the magazines? If you can find something positive about them, Laura will be more receptive to your opinions about the models and expensive clothes. Being open to Laura's interests will show her you accept and respect her judgment, even if you don't share all her tastes. She'll form a more balanced view if she also sees magazines that support diversity in body size and fashion. Look for some at your library or newsstand.*

4
Out of Bounds

Nature is forgiving. Just as
bodies adapt to deprivation, they respond
to healthy habits with renewed strength and power.

Two fourth graders called me for help on a school project. Their teacher had given them a case study involving a teenaged girl with a problem. "This girl needs to go on a diet," said one of the students. "She's overweight and out of shape. She puffs going up stairs. And she doesn't have a boyfriend."

I asked the height and weight of the teenager in the case study and realized—to the amazement of the fourth graders—the girl was already at a healthy weight. I gave the students suggestions for how their subject could increase her fitness and her self-esteem. And I attempted to explain that there isn't a connection between weight loss and boyfriends!

Everyone who *thinks* she should lose weight doesn't necessarily have a weight problem. Too many youngsters want to change their perfectly normal bodies. Some go to extremes to do so. A child at a healthy weight who thinks she has a weight problem actually has a body-image problem. And body-image problems can lead to real weight problems. It's enough to make a parent's head spin!

Like all complicated issues, weight and body-image concerns can be understood by breaking them down into manageable parts. That's what this chapter is about. Be assured that your child won't simply wake up one morning with a weight problem or an eating disorder: Kids gradually slip out of bounds. At any point, you can reach out and gently guide your child back within the boundaries of healthy living. The final four chapters of this book will show you how to do just that—or better still, prevent problems from developing in the first place. But first let's look at some of the complexities of body weight and body image.

Why Weight?

Parents fret about purple hair and body piercing, but the real problems begin when young people slip beyond the bounds of healthy, realistic body shapes. The pursuit of the perfect body has seven-year-olds dieting; preteens smoking; teenaged girls popping diet pills; teenaged boys gulping muscle-building drugs; girls *and* boys fasting and purging.

Throughout history, people have used everything from neck coils and neckties to corsets and elevator shoes to feel more attractive. Whether we like it or not, size counts—it always has. During times of scarcity, it's fashionable to be plump. In this present age of excess, you can't be too lean. Isn't it ironic that slim, well-toned bodies are the ideal at a time when so many of us are overly fat and out of shape?

Considering the reality of everyday life, the situation is hardly surprising. We motor to work and school (no time to walk!), and get so tired sitting at computers and battling traffic that we collapse in front of the TV at the end of the day. Many of us don't have enough time or energy to put food on the table—or even to wait for someone else to do it—so we seek shortcuts for shopping, cooking, eating, and cleaning up. Enter the purveyors of fast food to "do it all for you!" Lacing food with sugar and salt (no time to acquire a taste for something else!), they add plenty of fat to fill you up fast. It's easy to eat quickly and overshoot that "just right" amount when the servings are super-size! The food is inexpensive, too. Fast-food marketers don't miss a trick.

Desperate to reverse the effects of moving too little and eating too much, we direct $35 billion a year to North America's diet industry. Weight worries aren't restricted to adults, of course. Kids of all ages eat fast food, watch TV, use computers, ride instead of walk, and wear fashions designed for thin bodies. Often seen as a quick fix, dieting can harm children physically and emotionally. Weight-conscious kids don't think of that—or don't care. A U.S.-wide survey of 12,000 adolescents found 61 percent of girls and 28 percent of boys had been on a weight-loss diet within the last year. Other studies have shown that dieting is common in children as young as seven! Numerous studies of children's eating habits confirm a trend toward dieting among kids. At this rate, dieting could become "the norm!"

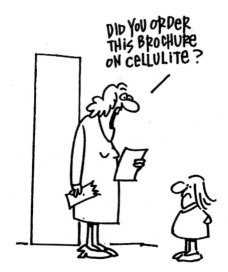

Tipping the Scales

The concept of "ideal" weights is outmoded. Today, the range of weights considered healthy is wider than ever. But this progressive thinking isn't reflected in the narrow standard of "physical correctness" that's become so fashionable. It's not politically correct to criticize people on the basis of age, race, gender, or ability, but it's okay to hassle them about their weight—apparently for their own good!

Many people who consider themselves health conscious are really "health anxious" when it comes to weight. The link between weight and health is tenuous, since fitness probably has a greater effect. There are risks associated with extremes in body weight at either end of the scale. The heaviest adults have a higher-than-average risk for heart disease, diabetes, and some types of cancer. Extremely thin people need to watch out for broken bones, complications from infections, and reproductive problems. Lifestyle—not weight—may be the greatest health determinant for most people who fall between the two extremes.

At what point does a child's weight affect her health? There are no clear-cut answers. Growth charts for kids, including Body Mass Index tables based on children's heights and weights, can be helpful in assessing risk. Lines drawn through growth charts categorize kids with the highest weight-to-height ratios as "overweight," while deeming those with the lowest weight-to-height ratios as "underweight." But some healthy kids don't conform to tables of averages, particularly if they're very muscular. Kids are generally taller today than children of previous generations. They also tend to have larger bones, more muscle, and proportionately more fat. That all adds up to more pounds of body weight.

Although it's difficult to say how much weight is too much for a given child, studies suggest that about 20 percent of today's kids have weight-related abnormalities in blood pressure, blood cholesterol, and insulin. Some heavy kids have problems breathing, especially when they're lying down. That can interfere with normal activities, including sleep. Kids with higher-than-average levels of body fat also reach puberty at younger-than-average ages. Girls can find themselves with breasts and periods long before they're ready to leave childhood. The general trend toward earlier sexual maturation is also linked with higher rates of teenage pregnancy and an increased risk of breast cancer (due to longer-term exposure to estrogen).

The emotional consequences of being larger than average may disturb children more than the physical risks. Kids learn that it's better to be slim than heavy everywhere they look—even at home. Parents worry about their own weights *and* their children's weights. Often parents are particularly troubled when daughters are large for their age and sons, small. One mom I know used to coax her slim eight-year-old boy to eat more. She was stunned when she glanced at one of his school notebooks and read, "My mother doesn't like the way I look."

Moms and dads instinctively want their kids to eat, but may send conflicting messages to larger-than-average children: "Eat, eat ... but not too much!" Even preschoolers make the connection between "fattening" food and body weight.

Do "obese" children become obese adults? Some do and some don't—and the reasons for the differences aren't clearly understood. During some developmental phases, kids may be temporarily fatter than usual. This commonly happens around a child's first birthday. During early childhood, kids tend to lose their "baby fat" so that by the time they're six, they seem to be all legs and arms! A child's fat levels will begin climbing shortly after that, peaking in the preteen years in preparation for the adolescent growth spurt. All of these growth cycles are "normal." But studies do show that when fat levels begin to increase at an earlier-than-usual age—at five, for example, rather than at six or seven—a child is more likely to become fatter than average. The longer a child is heavy during childhood, the more likely she'll continue to be heavy during her teens and into adulthood.

It's not easy to determine how much a person should weigh, especially during childhood. Adults with stable body weights know when they've gained or lost weight by comparing any changes to their "usual" weights. Because kids' and teens' bodies are constantly changing, "usual" weights don't exist. Weight gain is part of normal growth and development.

Despite their limitations, growth charts for kids can be helpful in tracking a child's weight in comparison to height, over time. The resulting pattern is a simple indicator of whether a child is growing consistently. Children who are meant to be tall and slim, short and stocky, or any other combination of traits, usually show that tendency in their weight-to-height ratio during early childhood.

Parents are just as concerned when babies and young children put on too *little* weight as too *much*. Some kids are naturally slimmer than average. As long as they follow a steady growth pattern, they're likely to be healthy. But if your child stops gaining weight, or if she loses weight, it's important to see your family doctor. While the rate at which a child gains weight slows down naturally during some stages, weight *loss* is always a concern because it signals an interruption in growth and development.

Weight is more sensitive than height to small deviations from regular eating and activity. When a child eats too little, she may stop gaining weight while continuing to grow in height, at least initially. If she goes back to eating normally, she may gain weight at a faster rate and resume her earlier growth curve for weight. This "catch-up" growth often occurs after a temporary setback such as an illness. But after a while, if a child's weight gain is slower than it should be—whether due to eating too little, or a digestive or metabolic problem—her growth in height may also be affected. Doctors call this "failure to thrive."

When kids eat too much—or don't get enough active play—their growth curve for weight can rise faster than their growth curve for height. A sudden, dramatic change in habits can cause a weight curve to spike upward. This happened with a four-year-old whose

mother fell into a deep depression after the breakup of her mar-
riage. The mother retreated to her couch and began to overeat,
and her daughter copied the behavior. The little girl's weight-to-
height ratio increased significantly over a year, and she became
extremely heavy. In a situation like that, if the family is able to
make some healthy lifestyle changes, the child may be able to stop
gaining extra weight. She may even "grow into" her weight.

Do We Have a Problem?

If you suspect your child is gaining too little or too much weight,
see your doctor or public health nurse. It's especially helpful if
your health-care provider measures your child's height and weight
at regular visits to help you monitor her growth rate. Be reassured
if her height and weight charts indicate she's growing consistently, even if she's smaller or larger than other children her age.
If there *is* a problem, growth records can indicate when your child
began to go off track, which will help the doctor make a diagnosis
and recommendations.

A medical condition can cause a child to gain too little or too
much weight. There may be a problem digesting food, absorbing
nutrients, or balancing hormones. A child may have a bowel
disorder, intestinal infection, or food sensitivity that interferes
with her growth, or she may have inherited a condition such
as the very rare Prader-Willi Syndrome, which causes excessive
weight gain.

Diabetes can also affect a child's weight. Children with Type 1
diabetes require insulin injections balanced by a regular routine
of eating and exercise. Type 1 diabetes results when the pancreas
isn't able to produce enough insulin, the substance that allows
body cells to absorb sugar. A child may lose weight when her body
doesn't have enough insulin and her blood-sugar levels are high.
Sadly, teenagers with diabetes often avoid taking their insulin in

an attempt to lose weight, putting themselves at risk for long-term complications such as kidney failure, circulatory problems, and blindness. (If you find that incredible, consider this: One study showed that some women expressed a willingness to give up five years of their lives if they could reach their preferred weight!)

Type 2 diabetes results when the pancreas still functions but doesn't produce enough insulin. Previously called "adult onset" diabetes, Type 2 diabetes has raised alarms because it's become increasingly common among children, perhaps due to today's lifestyle habits and higher body weights.

Your family doctor may refer your child to a pediatrician to help identify a possible weight problem and rule out any medical conditions. If the doctor diagnoses a weight problem with no immediate medical concerns, take some time to consider the options that might best serve your child. Don't look for a quick solution—it may do more harm than good. For many larger- or smaller-than-average children who *are* developing normally, real problems begin when their parents decide "something has to be done." Children can lose their natural ability to respond to signals of hunger and satisfaction when well-meaning parents and doctors impose outside controls on their eating.

It's important to remember that a child with a weight problem hasn't done anything "wrong." She may have inherited traits that affect her body shape. Her family's eating and activity habits may also have influenced her growth. Guilt about eating may set her up for a lifetime of dieting—and misery. Obesity is hard on kids, but it's harder still to feel loved less because of it.

Family counseling can be helpful when a child has a weight problem. This doesn't mean the family is "to blame." It simply means the lifestyles of others in the household usually affect a child's eating, activity, and relaxation. Singling out a child for treatment may make her feel bad about herself. Anything that lowers a child's self-esteem can worsen a weight-related problem.

A recent study showed that treating childhood obesity was more effective when parents attended a program *without* their kids. Parents learned to change family eating and activity patterns, and everyone benefited. The overweight kids in this study had greater success meeting their goals than kids treated directly in other programs. Researchers were correct in assuming overall changes in family habits would affect kids' behavior. Best of all, children were spared the feeling that they had a personal problem that needed "fixing."

Nutritionist Ellyn Satter suggests that treatment programs should identify and correct those aspects of a child's environment that may have triggered the abnormal weight gain or loss. It's not effective—or humane—to simply change a child's eating and activity habits without understanding what was happening in her life at the time her weight went off the rails. Satter stresses the importance of trust—not only between parent and child, but in the child's inborn ability to regulate her eating. Some children aren't meant to be slim—and no treatment will make it happen. That doesn't mean they can't grow up healthy, strong, and self-assured.

A weight-control program should allow a child to continue to grow in height, while not putting on too much weight. That usually doesn't mean losing weight, because weight gain is part of normal growth. Despite the typical adolescent growth spurt, some heavy kids never "grow into" their weight. Healthy eating and regular activity may not make a child slim, but these lifestyle habits can help prevent a heavy child from becoming even heavier.

Unfortunately, traditional treatment approaches for large children sometimes focus on dieting and restrained eating—behaviors that can set kids up for a lifetime of gaining, losing, and regaining weight. Some programs include regimented exercise that turns kids off physical activity, further contributing to extra weight gain.

Leaving Normal

Dieting affects more than eating habits—it can upset every part of a child's daily routine. Chronic dieters are moody, easily distracted, and self-critical. They eat erratically, and when they "lose control," they feel guilty and down on themselves.

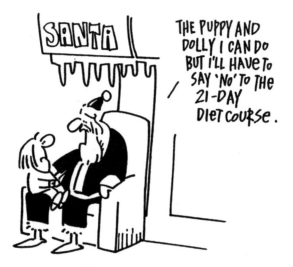

Never put your child on a diet. Diets are designed to override the body's natural signals to eat when hungry and stop when satisfied. Diets are based on the assumption that someone (let's call her Jane) usually eats too much, and someone else (let's call her Dr. Diet) knows just how much Jane *should* be eating. This assumption is faulty. First, Jane may already be at a healthy weight. Losing weight may compromise her health. Putting that aside for a moment, even if Jane appears to be overweight, she may be inactive rather than overeating. If Jane *is* overeating, how does Dr. Diet know exactly how much food she needs? All sorts of factors determine an individual's calorie needs. Chances are, Dr. Diet's advice is more of a hindrance than a help. Countless studies show 95 percent of dieters regain their lost weight, and then some.

When you eat less than usual, your body's natural instinct for survival kicks in, doing everything it can to get back on track. Hunger pains signal the need for fuel. The mind is distracted by thoughts of food and eating. Dieters are often so preoccupied with food that they lose interest in work, activity, sex, and companionship. The body's insistent plea for food makes it harder and harder to focus on anything else, so the dieter feels frustrated and irritable. If this is painful for adults, imagine how it feels for children!

In the honeymoon phase at the beginning of a diet, a person may lose a few pounds, but the body soon rallies its defenses—adjusting its metabolism to slow down weight loss. Inevitably, the dieter is driven to resume regular eating. When she does, she readily regains the lost weight—and sometimes more. Kids are subject to the same thwarted efforts as adult dieters—but with a further complication. All bodies need food to function and repair tissues, but *growing* bodies also need materials for expansion. Plenty of protein, minerals, and vitamins are needed to build bone, muscle, blood, organs, and nerves.

Because staying alive is the body's first priority, food that's in short supply is used to meet energy needs rather than build new tissue. Children who don't get enough to eat are small for their age—and sometimes never reach their full growth potential. A child with a stocky build can end up even shorter and heavier than if she'd been allowed to reach the height Nature intended for her. Dieting can impair the growth and development of every system of a child's body. Once a child is starving—as happens with some eating disorders—it's not a simple task to bring her back to a well-nourished state.

Even moderate and occasional dieting will take your child's attention away from her inner body signals to less reliable cues to eat. "Restrained eating" is something many kids learn from adults. Contrary to popular opinion, it isn't a healthy practice.

Restrained eaters are constantly watching their step around food. They trust outside influences—books, magazines, diet experts—more than they trust their bodies' signals for hunger and satisfaction. They adopt rules for eating based on simplistic, erroneous principles: "The fewer bad foods I eat, the better I am." "Going without food makes me a good, well-disciplined person." Or: "I just ate a couple of hours ago—I shouldn't be hungry again."

Parents sometimes try to restrain a child's eating because they want to "help" control her weight. Moms and dads usually mean well, but they can contribute to the very problem they hope to prevent. Comments such as "Do you *really* need another bun?" or "You've eaten enough," often prompt a child to eat secretly, which in turn makes her feel guilty about eating. In this situation, it's easy for a child to become preoccupied with food and eat in an out-of-control manner when she's away from her parents.

Despite their vigilance, most restrained eaters eat just as much as normal eaters do over time—and sometimes more! They're more likely to binge because they're constantly hungry (think about how fast and how much you eat when you're very hungry). Studies show that restrained eaters overeat whenever they let down their guard. Almost anything can do it—happiness, sadness, fatigue, excitement, boredom. Restrained eaters also tend to overdo it when someone gives them "permission" to eat. Because they're out of touch with their body signals, they watch for signs that it's appropriate to eat. When investigators in one study tampered with a clock to give subjects the impression it was time for dinner, restrained eaters ate more than normal eaters did in the same situation.

Teaching your child to restrain her eating will put her on a course of feast or famine. As Ellyn Satter says, kids start out as normal eaters. They eat when they're hungry and stop when they've had enough. Sometimes they eat more because the food tastes especially good. Sometimes they don't eat enough. On average, they eat about the same amount from one day to the next.

Normal eaters enjoy food, but they don't think about it constantly. Unfortunately, the pressure to be thin, coupled with the prevalence of dieting, means more and more kids are "leaving normal" at an alarming rate.

When body-fat levels drop too low, girls experience interruptions in their menstrual cycles—one of the ways in which Nature protects poorly nourished women from reproducing. Missing periods may seem convenient, but it's not healthy. A girl who's not menstruating can lose a measurable amount of bone after only a few months.

Experts suggest that dieting among boys is underreported. Because restrained eating is so common among girls, boys often consider it "feminine" and hesitate to talk about it. Among boys *and* girls, anti-diet messages are driving some dieting behavior underground. "No Diet Day" and similar public education initiatives are changing the way people talk about dieting—but they don't always change what people do. Kids who realize it's not acceptable to go on a diet may simply claim to eat nutritionally or to reject junk food. A sudden interest in vegetarian meals may also be a smoke screen for dieting or an eating disorder. These kids aren't being devious: They're adopting behaviors that society accepts and reinforces. Knowing that their actions may speak louder than their words, we need to pay close attention to how our kids eat—and how they live their lives.

Crossing the Line

It's easy to see how dieting can lead to an eating disorder. Current studies suggest that dieting can disturb the balance of brain chemicals—which can lead to binge eating. While dieting doesn't necessarily cause eating disorders, eating disorders rarely occur without dieting as a first step. Abnormal eating can be seen as a continuum from restrained eating all the way to a full-fledged eating disorder. Some children put themselves on that path before they even reach their teens.

Sadly, eating disorders are about more than eating: They affect how a child feels about herself, how she relates to others, and how she spends her time. Eating disorders are serious. Sometimes they're fatal. The most common type is bulimia nervosa, which affects an estimated one to five percent of kids. Young people with bulimia may have normal weights and appear to be healthy, but they binge at least twice a week and later try to compensate by vomiting or taking laxatives. Lots of kids consider vomiting an "easy way out" when they feel they've eaten too much. Little do they know how much physical and emotional damage lies ahead if it becomes a habit.

A person with bulimia will likely isolate herself from her family and social group. Regular self-induced vomiting requires privacy. And like anyone else who feels guilty about overeating, a person with bulimia tends to do her binge eating alone. Bulimia can be expensive, challenging its victim to find the cash to purchase large amounts of food. Some resort to stealing money or food.

The second most common eating disorder is anorexia nervosa, a condition in which a person desires, above all else, to be pencil slim. High achievers and perfectionists, girls and boys with anorexia see their bodies in a distorted way. They often consider themselves to be too fat, even when their bodies are skeletal. They diet obsessively, exercise compulsively, and sometimes purge. Anorexia nervosa strikes an estimated two to 10 people per 1,000, most of them girls and young women. Eating disorders affect some groups of people in disproportionate numbers: An estimated one in five athletes and dancers suffers from this condition. More than one person of every six with anorexia nervosa will die of its effects.

Consider how it would feel to wake up inside the skin of someone with anorexia. You might take a quick shower, then look at yourself in the mirror. You feel uneasy if you can pinch a little flesh around your stomach. If the numbers on the bathroom scale are low, they must be wrong. You decide to skip breakfast. You don a heavy sweater because you always feel cold. You comb your hair and watch as some falls onto the dresser. Maybe your dad hassles you about eating. You tell him you can't eat before gym class. You peek at the lunch your mom packed, deciding to keep the salad and apple, but dump the cheese sandwich and salad dressing because the feeling of fat in your mouth revolts you. You save the apple until after school, so you won't be too hungry at dinner. You go for a run when the rest of the family eats so your parents won't watch every bite. Even though several assignments are due, you *must* make time for your run. You wonder as you go to school if your butt looks fat in your jeans. Your friends said they looked cool, but you had wanted them one size smaller. Then, you would have looked *perfect*.

People with anorexia don't think they have a problem. It's not surprising, really. When they lose the first few pounds, we say they look great and ask how they did it. We compliment them on their "willpower" and "discipline." Reality hits us later, when we realize their restrained eating is extreme and their exercise routine compulsive. We scorn their "sick" behavior, but it's too late. For someone with anorexia, weighing less and less just means she's getting "better."

People with bulimia know they have a problem. No one compliments you for hanging over a toilet bowl on a regular basis. While "conquering" hunger may make someone with anorexia feel in control, bingeing and vomiting do nothing to boost the self-esteem of a person with bulimia. She feels guilty when she binges and grossed out when she purges. Her throat is sore. Her tooth enamel is eroding from exposure to stomach acids. So why does she do it? She's afraid of being fat.

There are other types of eating disorders, all damaging to body and spirit. Binge eating disorder is a term applied to conditions that don't meet the diagnostic criteria for either anorexia or bulimia.

Sometimes people chew and spit out large quantities of food. Sometimes they binge without purging, apparently indifferent to their weight or shape. In reverse anorexia—found especially in male weight lifters—a person feels too small, despite being average or above average in weight and muscle definition.

Don't get caught up in terminology. The line between these different types of eating disorders is often blurred. It takes a health professional with special training to make a diagnosis. But knowing the signs and symptoms of eating disorders can alert you to what's happening to a child before dangerous practices become habits. Young people who show signs of abnormal eating and activity need counseling. Privacy and confidentiality are essential. At school, rumors about eating disorders spread quickly, making sufferers feel isolated and defensive.

Spotting Signs of an Eating Disorder

The following signs, alone or in combination, can signal a disturbed eating pattern or self-image.

Be alert to a child's complaining about feeling fat. Watch for changes in behavior, such as skipping meals or eating alone. Keep an eye out for lost body fat, and signs of water retention such as puffiness around the joints.

Weight loss and muscle wasting can cause weakness, cramps, fatigue, lethargy, dizziness, hair loss, and increased sensitivity to cold. Moodiness and depression are common, as are constipation and menstrual irregularities.

Compulsive exercising and perfectionist, ritualistic habits are typical of some eating disorders. A child may use the bathroom often, especially after meals. Tooth discoloration can signify loss of enamel from vomiting.

Laxative abuse can cause iron-deficiency anemia and rectal bleeding.

If you're worried, talk to a counselor or nutritionist familiar with eating disorders. Don't jump to conclusions: Only a professional can diagnose an eating disorder. It's natural to feel uncertain about whether a problem exists—but it's also important not to delay getting help.

It's important to include families in counseling a child with a suspected eating disorder, but parents shouldn't try to cope without outside help. Moms and dads can't be therapists and all-important supporters at the same time. Highly trained professionals, including mental-health counselors, doctors, and dietitian/nutritionists often work as a team to help people with disturbed eating understand what's wrong and take corrective action. This is a problem that goes well beyond eating. It's essential that all team members be knowledgeable about eating disorders, and that there be one key therapist available for regular advice. Getting "well" isn't a quick process, mentally or physically. Someone with anorexia who has experienced extreme weight loss needs a dietitian's supervision to *gradually* reestablish a normal eating pattern and regain weight. Starvation disturbs the body's metabolism and fluid balance. "Shocking" a starved body with food and nutrients can result in seizures and death.

There's no shame in getting off track—but it *is* a shame to let a young person struggle alone with a problem that affects every aspect of day-to-day living in what everyone says are the "best years" of her life. Eating disorders can be treated, but imagine how much pain and suffering *prevention* could avoid! Despite the widespread incidence of dieting, the "never say diet" message is catching on. Unfortunately, teaching kids that dieting is both ineffective and unpleasant isn't enough to deter them from the illusive goal of physical perfection. What if more of us appreciated the wonderful diversity of human beings? What if more kids dared to let their natural weight evolve through healthy eating and exercise? It can happen if we let it.

Risky Business

It's tough to stick to diets and demanding exercise regimens. Is it any wonder so many of us look for a way to make it a little easier? The desire to be slim is one of the motivating factors on which the tobacco industry capitalizes. Although many adults have quit smoking, young girls represent a growing market. It's easy to see why. Magazine ads show skinny models holding cigarettes branded "slim" and "cool." Tobacco companies regularly sponsor fashion shows. Novelties such as flavored cigarettes—even more concentrated in nicotine and tar than regular cigarettes—are a hit with young smokers. And, thwarted by tougher regulations for print and TV advertising, tobacco companies have turned to the Internet to reach potential consumers.

The U.S. National Cancer Institute says that people who start to smoke when they're kids are likely to face a greater risk of lung cancer than those who start later. Smoking is one of the most health-damaging habits known to medical science and, contrary to what some smokers believe, it's not an effective weight-control method. Because nicotine speeds up the metabolism, smokers usually put on a few pounds when they quit. Those who resume smoking tend not to drop the extra weight. The average smoker isn't usually any slimmer than the average nonsmoker. Sadly, the more weight a smoker gains, the more cigarettes she may have to smoke to get her usual hit of nicotine.

Nicotine isn't the only drug that tempts people desperate to lose weight. Diet pills have been around for generations—the earliest ones contained cyanide! Thirty years ago, amphetamine was the diet drug of choice. Aptly referred to as "speed," it's available today in "Ecstasy" and other street drugs. Young and old, users eager to lose a little weight suffer jangled nerves and risk high blood pressure, heart problems, and death.

The diet pills dispensed by your neighborhood pharmacist may not be any safer. In the late 1990s, dexfenfluramine was yanked off the market after one in four users developed leaky heart valves. Another diet pill of dubious effectiveness was approved for sale a year later. Despite the risks, the search goes on for a magic bullet to melt away those unwanted pounds.

While girls try to whittle themselves down to shadows, boys try to emulate role models with washboard abs and humungous upper bodies. The effort can make gym workouts a full-time job! Are there any shortcuts? Enter protein powders and muscle-enhancing chemicals.

Perhaps due in part to the blurred line between amateur and professional sport, it's not unusual for Olympic athletes to be disqualified for drug use. It's accepted that professional athletes use performance- and muscle-enhancing drugs, and hardly surprising when kids in training follow suit. After St. Louis Cardinals' slugger Mark McGwire admitted to using androstenedione when he set a new world record for home runs, the drug's use in Canada reportedly increased seven-fold.

Boys who pump iron in the basement or hang out at neighborhood gyms spend big bucks on everything from protein powders to dangerous steroids, all in the pursuit of "getting big." Kids talk openly about the side effects of steroids—acne, hair loss, shrunken testicles, depression, and "steroid rages" in which normally mild-mannered guys fly off the handle. Like many street drugs, black-market steroids are often "cut" with other chemicals. Why risk so much to look "ripped"? Ask, and you'll get the age-old answer: to attract girls, and win the respect of other guys.

It's not a pretty picture: teens smoking, throwing up, taking drugs, picking fights. But there *are* alternatives. Parents and teachers can help kids find healthier ways to cope with peer pressures and feel good about themselves. You and your children can learn to eat in response to your own body signals. You can make time for play and active living. You can like yourself—and accept your body—while striving to be fit and strong. This is already a way of life for millions of people attuned to Nature's lessons. *Every* child deserves the chance to thrive. The next chapters will show you how to help *your* child do just that.

Because You Asked about Weight and Body Image

Q: My two-year-old son Sean is always hungry. He's such an eager eater that we feel it's necessary to limit his food intake. But now, Sean tries to sneak food when our backs are turned. My husband ate too much as a kid and his overweight teen years were unhappy.

A: *I suggest you and your husband discuss Sean's eating habits with a dietitian. See your doctor first to rule out any health problems, and get a referral. It sounds as if Sean is still hungry after eating what you've provided, so it's natural for him to want to help himself when your backs are turned. In general, toddlers are less likely to gain excess weight when they're free to eat the amount they want at regular meal and snack times than when their parents impose outer controls. With guidance from a dietitian, offer Sean a variety of wholesome foods and allow him to follow his appetite. Having been restricted, he may overdo it at first, but once he realizes he can satisfy his hunger, his overeating should abate.*

Q: My preschooler is chubby. She just loves to eat, especially mashed potatoes and gravy and all sorts of sweets. If I let her serve herself at the table, she scoops huge servings of potatoes or pasta onto her plate!

A: *Your daughter may or may not be overeating. Commenting on the amount of food she takes will only make her feel bad—and perhaps force her to pilfer food. Do continue to let her serve herself, but fill your serving dishes with just enough food for the whole family. Encourage everyone to share, without singling her out. There should be enough so no one leaves the table hungry. Mashed potatoes are a nourishing food, but it'll be healthier for everyone if you offer them occasionally (unless you make them with skim milk powder and potato water, and skip the gravy). I'd like to see you limit the number of sweets you bring into the house, too. When you offer your child foods that aren't so high in fat and sugar, you'll feel more comfortable when she eats with gusto. Speak privately (not in front of your daughter) to a doctor, public health nurse, or dietitian about your concerns.*

Q: My 12-year-old son and nine-year-old daughter are skinny, just like my husband. They eat a lot of junk food, but they seem to be pretty healthy. They don't like sports, but I don't think it matters since it's unlikely they'll ever have a weight problem. Should I get on their case?

A: *Nagging never works, does it? Do try to make it easy for your kids to eat well by having healthy snacks ready to serve and limiting the "junk" food in the house. Not all children are athletes, but all kids—regardless of weight—benefit from plenty of active play. A slim child needs wholesome food and enjoyable exercise as much as any other kid. Please take to heart the guidelines for healthy living in the following chapters.*

Q: Our teenaged son is taking a supplement called "creatine phosphate." He's convinced it will help him "bulk up." Is he wasting his money? More importantly, is this supplement harmful?

A: *I'd prefer a future in which kids exercise and eat well rather than take supplements they don't need. If your son's determined, however, this is what you need to know. Creatine is a natural compound that the body produces to metabolize food energy. It's also found in meat, fish, and poultry. Used as a supplement, it appears to speed up muscles' recovery time for activities such as weight lifting or sprinting that require brief, intense effort. It's expensive—and the jury's still out on its long-term consequences. Encourage your son to go off creatine every few months for at least a month. A recent study showed creatine levels in skeletal muscle returned to normal 28 days after the supplement was discontinued.*

Q: We're beside ourselves with worry about our 18-year-old daughter. Her weight has dropped from 135 pounds (61 kg) to 95 pounds (43 kg). She's an exercise fanatic and refuses to eat anything that contains fat. We've begged her to go to the doctor, but she says she's never felt better. Despite what she says, she's an emotional wreck and so are we.

A: *Tell your daughter that you love her and that her eating and exercise habits have you worried. Don't mention "eating disorders" or try to diagnose the problem. Call your local mental-health center or family doctor and make an appointment for the family. If your daughter refuses to attend, go anyway. You're right to be concerned.*

PART II

"E"-sy Growing

5
The Art of Eating

*Nature speaks to us softly. If we
listen, we know when our bodies need
food—and when we've taken enough.*

We all want our children to eat well. But where do we begin to teach them how? With 40,000 different products at the super-market—and new ones introduced daily—we've never been more confused about what to put into our mouths. Food can be a tonic or a toxin; eating the high point of the day or a nuisance.

In some ways, we've become detached from food. Most of us don't grow our own and many don't know or care where food comes from. The cooking channel makes for entertaining televi-sion, but do we really jot down the recipes? Surveys claim that many of us spend only 15 to 30 minutes a day cooking. Neverthe-less, we worry. While bright signs beckon us to drive in and eat up, the evening paper says we're digging our graves with our knives and forks.

As parents, we probably worry too much. I've seen ideas about feeding kids come and go, but despite changes in nutritional advice over the years, the importance of regular, mindful eating remains undisputed. There will always be new scientific reports telling us *what* to eat, but Nature also shows us *how* to eat. This chapter will help you reclaim the art of eating, while keeping the science in perspective. Stay with me through each stage as I show you how to help your child develop a positive relationship with food, one step at a time. I'll focus here on *how* to eat, and save the specifics of *what* to eat for the next chapter.

Back to Basics

As a parent, there's plenty you can do to ensure that your child's relationship with food is healthy and positive, right from the start.

We know that bodies need constant nourishment, especially when they're young and growing. This makes eating regularly—four to six times a day—very important. You can do your part by establishing regular meal and snack times. But remember the rule of shared responsibility: Always let your child decide if he's hungry, and if so, how much to eat. Practicing this healthy habit will help your child stay in tune with his appetite. It will help him eat the amount that's right for him, now and throughout his life. It's an essential step on the way to a healthy, natural body weight.

You can expect a child who follows his appetite to eat more on some occasions, and less on others. One day, he may eat heartily at breakfast and the next, toy with his breakfast but eat more lunch. Despite these variations, kids usually eat, on average, about the same number of calories each day.

Like most kids, your child will sometimes ask for food when he's not really hungry. A toddler who suddenly spots candy at the store may want to eat it on the spot. Calmly say "no" and move on, helping him focus his attention on something else. A preschooler curious about your evening guests may get out of bed, claiming to be hungry. Ask, "Are you *really* hungry, or would you like to sit with us awhile?" Chances are, he'll be happy to sit for 10 minutes or so and then head back to bed. Provide your child with a dependable but flexible routine. You wouldn't want him to eat candy every time he sees it, but that doesn't mean it should never pass his lips! And while hunger shouldn't be a regular excuse to get up at night, an occasional unscheduled snack won't hurt.

When kids *are* hungry, they need enough time to eat and their bodies need enough time to register that they've had enough. Your child's body will "shout" when it's hungry and "whisper" when it's satisfied. Eating on the run makes it hard to pick up on these subtle cues. How much time is enough? That depends on the child and the circumstances. Most kids need at least 15 minutes to eat a meal. Don't expect much more when your child's in a hurry to go out and play. If the whole family is gathered for pleasant conversation, however, 30 minutes or more may be appropriate.

The "right space" can help a child hone his eating skills. Dining at a table with family or friends is more conducive to conscious, purposeful eating than grabbing a bite on the run or mindlessly munching in front of the TV. But the right space is more than a physical place—it's an environment in which a child is free to learn by trial and error, and by following the example of others. Create a nurturing place where your child can gain confidence and come to associate good food with good times—a place where people come first, and food is secondary!

Making a Beautiful Baby

When you're pregnant, your developing baby will share everything you put into your mouth—and every experience you encounter. Your weight gain will affect your child's birth-weight, which in turn will affect his health. It's important to gain enough to nourish your baby, but you won't want to make it too difficult to get your figure back after the baby arrives.

During pregnancy, expect a steady weight gain that begins slowly and speeds up in the weeks before birth. The pattern of weight gain is as important as the number of pounds or kilos you gain. Between 25 and 35 pounds (11.5 to 16 kg) is a healthy average weight gain. Depending on your pre-pregnancy weight and whether you're carrying more than one developing baby, your doctor may encourage you to gain more or less.

Plan to give yourself about a year to get back to your pre-pregnancy shape. Trying to lose weight too quickly after your baby's birth can affect the production of breast milk.

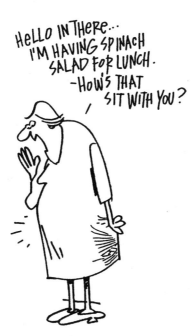

HeLLO IN THeRe...
I'M HAVING SPINACH
SALAD FOR LUNCH.
-HOW'S THAT
SIT WITH YOU?

The Infant – Life after Birth

Babies cry when they're hungry and relax when they've had enough to eat. Of course, babies cry for other reasons, too—which can be hard on new parents! As you and your baby become well acquainted, you'll learn to better understand each other. Your baby will do his part by letting you know when he's hungry—and you'll do yours by recognizing his hunger and feeding him promptly.

Breastfeeding can be a wonderful bridge between prenatal life and early childhood. Vancouver physician and author Gabor Maté refers to the breastfeeding period as "the second nine months of gestation." Breastfeeding, in fact, is a good model for how to eat. A mother offers her child the best possible food, and he takes the amount he needs, while the physical closeness between mother and babe creates the "right space" for pleasurable eating. A few words of caution: In the early days, when you're still learning to interpret your baby's signals, try to avoid feeding him every time he fusses. Feeding on demand may seem like a natural response, but it can actually make life more confusing for both of you. You won't learn to figure out when he's *really* hungry—and he'll get the idea that he should eat every time he feels uncomfortable.

Making Mother's Milk

During pregnancy, a woman's breasts—regardless of size—become busy construction sites as dozens of ducts and small saclike containers called "alveoli" get ready to produce milk. Birth triggers a sudden dramatic change in Mom's hormones. Levels of estrogen and progesterone drop, while the pituitary gland starts making plenty of the hormone "prolactin." The crucial next step is for the baby to suck at the breast. Nerves beneath the skin surrounding the nipple send a message to the brain that directs the pituitary gland to release prolactin, which stimulates the alveolar cells to make milk. "Colostrum"—a special fluid rich in nutrients and antibodies—is the first substance the breasts secrete. It's all a baby needs during the first few days before his mother's milk "comes in" and she starts producing an appreciable amount. The pituitary gland also releases a hormone called "oxytocin," which stimulates the contraction of breast cells and helps the milk move through the duct system and into the baby's mouth. This process is called "let-down." If a mom breastfeeds right after delivery, oxytocin also stimulates the contraction of her uterus, helping to stop the bleeding. Minor emotional upsets and stresses can affect oxytocin levels. Small changes in circulating oxytocin affect the let-down reflex, making it hard for a mom to breastfeed when she's upset.

You probably know that breast milk is good for babies, but you may not have considered all the advantages of breastfeeding your own infant. Apart from providing your baby with excellent nutrition, your breast milk can protect him from ear and respiratory infections, diarrhea, and anemia, as well as future problems such as allergies, asthma, diabetes, or excess weight. A recent German study showed that the longer a mother breastfeeds before introducing formula or solid food, the less likely her child will be to gain excess fat by age five or six. That result doesn't surprise me. After all, breastfed babies aren't coaxed to finish "the last little bit" as bottle-fed babies sometimes are.

Breastfeeding benefits you, too. Because the extra fat you stored late in pregnancy is used to produce milk, breastfeeding makes it easier to return to your pre-pregnancy weight. It may also reduce your risk of breast cancer. And there's no doubt you'll come out ahead financially—infant formula is expensive.

Learning to breastfeed isn't difficult, but like any "team activity," it requires instruction, coaching, and plenty of practice. It means learning how to relax, to calm your baby, to recognize when he's hungry, to position him to latch onto the breast properly, and to notice when he's had enough. Your baby is more likely to swallow comfortably and get enough milk with the right feeding technique (learn how to burp him so he won't feel gassy). Proper positioning can also help prevent sore nipples or a breast infection.

When I had my first child over 20 years ago, I stayed in hospital for nearly a week, getting plenty of help with breastfeeding. Today, many new moms are sprung in 24 hours or less! Before you leave the hospital, ask for the name of a lactation consultant or public health nurse who can help you learn good techniques. An experienced friend can also help.

When you first start to breastfeed, both you and your baby will have a full-time job on your hands (forget about all those things you were going to do on your maternity leave!). A newborn may be hungry every hour or two. During the first few weeks after birth, his frequent sucking will help establish your milk supply, which is why I don't recommend giving your breastfeeding baby a pacifier or bottle at first—it's more helpful for him to do all his sucking at the breast. Once you're making plenty of milk, however, you may want to give your baby an occasional bottle—preferably filled with pumped breast milk.

A breastfed baby needs his mom to get plenty of fluids, good nutrition, rest, and relaxation so she'll be able to make enough milk. He'll be affected by cigarette smoke, alcohol, and caffeine if Mom doesn't continue to avoid these substances as she did during pregnancy.

While many moms find breastfeeding satisfying, life as a walking, talking, 24-hour snack bar is exhausting! Don't hesitate to ask for help with the baby and household—and some moral support, as well. If you're going to feed your baby often—and still have a life—you'll want to feel okay about breastfeeding whenever and wherever your baby gets hungry. Thankfully, more people are realizing that we all have a responsibility to help moms feel comfortable about breastfeeding in public.

Despite its many benefits, breastfeeding isn't for everyone. It's important to respect a woman's decision about what's best for her and her baby. While some women simply choose not to breastfeed, others face health problems that make it inappropriate.

If you have difficulty producing enough milk, ask your doctor or nurse for advice. You may only need some extra coaching. However, a very small number of mothers really *can't* make enough milk, and the cause is beyond their control. If you find yourself in this situation, don't feel guilty or inadequate. The best way to get around the problem and help your baby thrive is to supplement your own milk with a commercially prepared infant formula. You don't need to stop breastfeeding—just offer your baby some formula after you've nursed him. He may do fine with this "topping up," or he may begin nursing less and taking more from the bottle, eventually giving up breastfeeding altogether. Either way, you can continue to snuggle your baby as you feed him, reassuring him with your closeness. Technique is important with bottle feeding, too. Ask a nurse to show you how to minimize the amount of air your baby swallows, and how to burp him after feeding. Never prop a bottle for your baby—he may aspirate some of the contents.

While it's healthy for a child to eat regularly, there is a downside to eating *too* often. A baby's teeth can begin to decay if he sips milk or juice too frequently, or nods off with a nipple in his mouth, the liquid pooling around his teeth. This condition is called "nursing bottle" syndrome, but dozing at the breast can cause it, too. Breast milk and formula both contain sugar. Protect your baby's teeth by putting him to bed after he's completely finished nursing, and by not sending him to bed with a bottle. Of course, dental hygiene is important, too: As soon as your baby's teeth erupt, wipe them with a soft cloth after each feeding. Your dentist or dental hygienist can help you care for your baby's teeth right from the start.

The Older Baby - One of the Family

Mom brushes a nipple against her infant's cheek, and he latches on. As your baby gets older, he'll need only to see the nipple to take it into his mouth. When it's time for solid food, the same principle applies. Provided he's hungry, a child faced with a spoonful of food will open his mouth and close his lips over the spoon. Whether nursing or spoon-feeding, it's important to maintain eye contact with your baby so he can let you know when he wants more and when he wants to stop eating. Smiling and speaking quietly to your baby can make mealtime a pleasant occasion, rather than a chore to get through quickly.

Babies don't like it when someone forces a nipple or spoon into their mouths—or sneaks it in by distracting them with something else. Would you? Imagine relaxing at a restaurant table when your friend suddenly gasps: "That's Tom Cruise!" As you turn to look, your mouth dropping open in surprise, in goes a spoon of mashed peas. You might trust your friend a little less after that! Yet, many

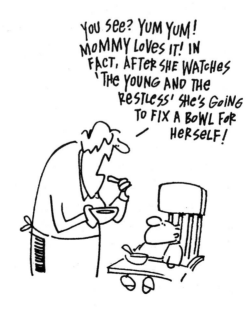

well-meaning parents try to trick their children into eating. Believe me: It's more comfortable for everyone if the baby is allowed to see the spoon coming. If he clamps his mouth shut and jerks his head away, his refusal should be respected. His body is telling him he's had enough.

At around six months of age, your baby may be able to sit up (with a little help), take food from a spoon, use his tongue to push the food to the back of his mouth, and swallow. Your baby may reach that developmental stage sooner—perhaps at four or five months—but he won't be ready for solid food until he does. Parents are often tempted to start solid food too soon, believing it will help babies sleep through the night. But infants younger than four months who seem to need more food are better off nursing for longer periods. That's because breast milk and formula are more concentrated in calories than a baby's first solid foods. If, however, an older baby *stops* sleeping through the night and seems hungry after nursing, he may be ready for more solids.

During the second six months of life, babies love to put everything into their mouths. They also tend to be more receptive than toddlers are to new foods and flavors. Don't miss this golden opportunity to introduce cereal, veggies, and other nourishing foods.

The introduction of solids allows an infant to move from sucking to spoon feeding, and from liquids to more textured foods. When he starts to chew, he'll need still more texture and will begin to accept lumpier foods. At this stage, he'll probably show an interest in holding the spoon himself and picking up pieces of food with his fingers—making safety a key concern. Always keep an eye on your baby while he's eating. Avoid foods that can cause choking, such as popcorn, raisins, and nuts. Chop foods such as grapes or meats—including wieners—into tiny pieces. Grate raw veggies (messy, but safe!). Never add infant cereal to a nursing bottle. Not only can it delay your baby's progress to more advanced eating skills, it also presents a potential choking hazard.

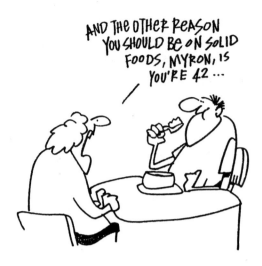

AND THE OTHER REASON YOU SHOULD BE ON SOLID FOODS, MYRON, IS YOU'RE 42 ...

Some babies nurse or take a bottle well into the second year or longer: The decision to wean is entirely up to you and your child. By the time their first birthdays roll along, many babies are eating a wide variety of family foods and drinking from a cup. They like to feed themselves, although transferring food to a spoon and getting it into that small opening under their noses is tricky! This is not the time to qualify for a Good Housekeeping Seal of Approval! Your baby will enjoy practicing his new skills more if you can tolerate some messiness at meals. (Tip: A plastic tarp under the high chair makes cleanup easier!)

You may be tempted to help your baby more than necessary—meals are quicker and tidier when parents wield the spoon! But the object isn't simply to get food into him. It's far more important to help him master the art of eating. As he does, he'll feel good about his growing independence and will look favorably upon mealtimes. That's a good trade-off for a little messiness in the kitchen!

As soon as he starts eating solid food, let your baby become a regular at the family table by coordinating his meals and snacks with yours. While you may wish to have an occasional "adults only" meal, everyone benefits when the older baby is included at most meals. By watching parents and siblings, babies learn a lot about eating and interacting with others.

The Toddler – Stepping Out

Toddlers are natural panhandlers. They're on the move and they know all about refrigerators and cookie cupboards! Is it any wonder that a mom sometimes takes the line of least resistance and throws crackers at her toddler while she tries to cook a meal? I've done it myself, but watch out! While regular eating is important, constant grazing can lead to overeating and tooth decay.

Toddlers need three regular meals a day with snacks in between—their little bodies can't go too long without eating. Provide your toddler with a booster seat that brings him up to a comfortable level at the table. Give him sturdy, nonbreakable cups, bowls, and plates that are heavy enough to resist spilling. A shallow bowl may make it easier for him to scoop up his food. Thick, short-handled spoons and forks are more manageable than adult-size cutlery. These little details can make the difference between a happy eater and a child who finds mealtime frustrating!

Restaurants that provide high chairs and booster seats are usually "child friendly." When you take your toddler out for dinner, it'll be more relaxing for everyone—family, servers, and other guests—if you plan to eat early before the "crowd" arrives. Keep your options open. Is it one of those days when your toddler wakes the baby and no one has an afternoon nap (again, I speak from experience)? It may be a good idea to reschedule that special dinner out.

Once in a while, your toddler will pester you for something he spots in the cupboard or at the grocery store. But deep down (sometimes *really* deep down!), he'll come to appreciate the security of your deciding what he can eat. You'll keep up your end of

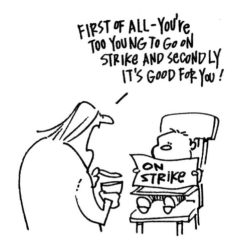

the bargain if you let him respond to his appetite: Occasionally he'll refuse food, and at other times he'll eat more than you anticipate. Assist him in helping himself from serving dishes, rather than putting a plate of food in front of him. Encourage him to take small amounts to begin with, and more if he's still hungry.

If other people sometimes take care of your child, be sure to explain his eating routine and ask for their cooperation in allowing him to follow his appetite. Many daycare and preschool leaders sit at the table with children, allowing them to serve themselves as they maintain a friendly, accepting atmosphere. Parents are often surprised at what their kids will eat at daycare or someone else's house, under the influence of other children! Some daycare centers and preschools also enrich their programs with cooking experiences and storybooks featuring wholesome food. Visit your local library for children's books that reinforce the eating habits you value.

While your child is still a toddler, encourage him to "help" in the kitchen. By letting him put the vegetables you've chopped into a pot or salad bowl, you'll give him a stake in eating the final product. If you'd like someday to have a teenager who helps with dinner, this is a good time to start training!

The Preschooler – Parents' Little Helper

Preschoolers pick up hundreds of words and ideas in a brief span of two or three years. They learn to socialize, play games, make things, and spend money. They develop strong bodies—and minds of their own.

Your preschooler may be a miniature lawyer with compelling arguments for getting a sugary snack. Or he may revert to throwing a tantrum, if that approach brought results when he was a toddler! Get your preschooler working *with* you instead of against you. Give him opportunities to use his ever-expanding skills. The three-year-old who's begging for a handout while you cook will stop fussing if you let him stand on a chair at the sink to wash the veggies (yes, you'll have to wipe up a little water afterward!). He'll be thrilled if you let him use a plastic knife to slice a banana for the fruit salad.

A four-year-old will enjoy the responsibility of setting the table, especially if he gets to decide on a suitable centerpiece (a small toy can be as attractive as a vase of flowers). Suppress your adult urge to "do it right" after he's done the job (show him how Mommy or Daddy does it by setting the table with him the first few times). He may also be ready to tear salad greens or put away the extra veggies in the refrigerator.

The versatile five-year-old can often remove the seeds from split sweet peppers, wash and spin lettuce, unload the lower level of the dishwasher onto the countertop (provided there are no sharp knives or overly fragile glasses and china), and clear the table. Of course, these are only suggestions. Be prepared to let your child surprise you with his capacity to be helpful!

Preschoolers love candles, especially if—under supervision—they get to blow them out at the end of the meal. They also delight in briefly holding hands around the table before the meal begins. Little rituals such as these help make mealtime fun and relaxing—a time to savor food and enjoy the company, rather than gobble and go.

As a preschooler, your child may catch you off guard with a sudden increase in appetite. Expect a growth spurt to follow. There will also be times when he grows slowly and doesn't seem as hungry as usual. When that happens, parents often panic and start to coax their child to eat. Fearing an eating problem, they create one! I've met moms at our kindergarten clinics who've resorted to spoon-feeding their five-year-olds. I remind them that force-feeding isn't a learning experience!

When a child enters a fussy phase, many a desperate parent becomes a short-order cook, catering to the child's limited appetite and tastes. Before long, Junior is eating in front of the TV most nights, demanding macaroni and cheese made from a box, while Mom or Dad cooks a "real meal" for the others. This can be the beginning of the end of family meals.

Parents need to stick together at times like this—even if they live in separate households. When parents fear their control is slipping away, it's easy for tension at the dinner table to become magnified out of all proportion. Maintain your cool *and* your long-term objectives! Coaxing, pleading, and insisting won't get your child to eat. Deciding to eat is his job—not yours. When kids aren't very hungry, they tend to be selective, so don't be surprised if your child wants to stick with his favorites during this phase.

Remember that choosing family foods is your job. I wouldn't routinely ask a preschooler what I should make for dinner, although I'd serve his favorite meal several times a month (if you're organized enough to have a monthly meal plan, you could let him slot his Number 1 choice into three or four meals). There are lots of ways to help a young child feel included while you remain in charge of meal planning. Offer him a choice between flat and curly noodles, for example. Or ask: "Would you like your carrots cooked or raw today?"

Whether or not your child goes through a finicky phase, avoid the temptation to link eating with body weight. Don't tell him he won't grow if he doesn't eat more food. Don't tell him he'll get too big if he eats too much. These thoughts may arise if you heard them yourself as a child, but these oversimplifications are just not true. They won't help your child eat well. In fact, they'll only make him feel uncomfortable about food and eating. If you think his eating may truly be abnormal, talk to your doctor or public health nurse without making your child aware of your fears.

The Primary School Child – A Taste of Independence

It's a little scary. We send our kids to school and things are never quite the same again. New authority figures and role models emerge ("You were right, Mom. My teacher says milk *is* good for me!"). They meet other kids who open their eyes to new possibilities ("Tara doesn't get an apple in her lunch. She gets little bags of candy made from squished-up fruit."). They go to friends' houses after school and come home with helpful suggestions ("Michael's mom makes popcorn in the microwave!").

When my kids started school, I let them pack their own lunches. I hate packing lunches and fortunately discovered early that youngsters consider it a privilege. By the time the novelty wears off, the habit's firmly formed! You don't have to make the lunch yourself in order to include an occasional surprise for your little student. It's easy to slip a small note, sticker, or cartoon strip into the bag when no one's looking.

Kids are less likely to throw away meals and snacks they've packed themselves. You can see what *is* left over if it comes home in reusable containers. Plastic containers with lids also save on paper waste (you'll need spares since they'll sometimes be forgotten at school). Help your kids make healthy choices by stocking a variety of nourishing foods. Chop extra veggies when you're cooking dinner so there's always a ready supply in the refrigerator. Offer a little guidance, too. (Otherwise, your first grader may head off to school with a piece of licorice, a cracker, and three bananas!)

When kids start school, they may have to eat at different times, and go longer between meals and snacks. Many also stay up too late watching TV and sleep too late to have breakfast. Time to prioritize! Regular eating (and plenty of rest) is essential to good health and active learning. Studies continue to show the importance of breakfast to school performance. Kids who don't "break the fast" each morning find it difficult to recall new material presented at school.

Check to ensure that your child has enough time to eat at school. Often schools provide lunchtime supervision for 15 minutes or less, then send the kids out to play. Sometimes children are so eager to play that *they're* the ones who decide to take a few bites and dash off to the playground! Some schools let the kids play first, then bring them back to eat during the last 15 minutes of the lunch period. This can work well as long as children who need a little more time to eat are permitted to finish their lunches after the bell rings.

The Preteen – Thinking Big!

Children in the upper elementary grades are great company—in and out of the kitchen. They combine the charm of early childhood with a capacity to think abstractly and an enthusiasm for new ideas. Concern about the environment may spur them to ask their parents to switch to reusable shopping bags. At home, they want to try foods they've had elsewhere. A child this age is open to what the world has to offer, but his parents' influence is still important.

Kids in the intermediate grades willingly embrace new experiences and responsibilities. They can't wait to grow up. If you let your child help with the shopping, he'll enjoy finding ways to "be green." Follow some of his new tips to minimize waste. School lessons may inspire him to eat more fresh, seasonal vegetables or switch from highly advertised cereals to less-processed products with simpler packaging. Kids in the upper elementary grades often have the analytical powers to see right through advertisements.

For many families, this is the time for the "big talk." Why not try regular, short, impromptu discussions instead? Don't forget to make the connection between sexual maturation and body image. Boys don't usually experience growth spurts until their early teens, but preteen girls often undergo dramatic physical changes. Girls need to know that it's healthy to put on a substantial amount of weight in the next few years—and that some of it will be fat. Many a preteen is aghast at the thought of fat rounding out her hips and breasts! It's an important time for moms to show open appreciation for normal, womanly bodies—including their own! Girls should be encouraged to follow their appetites since those who don't eat enough in the preteen years run the risk of stunting their height.

Kids this age are ready to cook and enjoy creating after-school snacks with their friends. Consider putting your child in charge of dinner once weekly, helping him follow the recipes. In no time, he'll be able to cook a real family meal with a little supervision. Parents sometimes ban their kids from the kitchen, fearing they'll hurt themselves or make a mess. That won't happen if you teach your child how to use equipment appropriate for his age and how to clean up properly. A 10-year-old may burn himself heating oil in a saucepan to make popcorn, but he can safely use a hot-air popper, even when he's alone in the kitchen.

The Young Teen – In Search of Self

It happens overnight. Middle-school children with their wide world-view suddenly narrow their focus right down to their own changing bodies. Weight and body-shape issues can become overwhelming. The young teenager who recently scoffed at fashion ads hears a tiny inner voice saying, "I want to look like that."

Young teens often begin to spend less time at home. They may bus to school, leaving early in the morning and getting home late in the afternoon. They may stay for after-school activities, too. If your child's world revolves around school, you may start to feel excluded.

Take heart. Studies show that parents still have substantial influence over young teenagers. Family meals are as important as ever: Kids need a safe haven where they can reflect on their feelings. Regular, healthy meals provide the physical and emotional security kids need, but young teens—with their many interests and commitments—often eat erratically. They're still child-like enough to eat too many sweets in one sitting, but "grown up" enough to try to make up for it by fasting after the feast! Skipping meals while gorging on snacks can wreak havoc with kids' equilibrium. Add wildly fluctuating blood-sugar levels to their raging hormones and you have a recipe for family conflict!

Do what you can to keep your child eating at the family table. It's too easy to lose touch with a teenager who gets into the habit of popping leftovers into the microwave and eating solo. Young teens commonly skip family meals and spend much of their time alone in their bedrooms. Kids who are involved in putting dinner on the table have a reason to come out of their rooms. Along with the added responsibility of helping, give your child some discretion in food choices and background music. If after-school activities make him late for dinner, delay family meals when possible so he can be included. Let your dining table be an island of sanity in your child's highly charged world!

The Older Teenager – No Fear of Flying!

The older teenager has one foot in your house and the other somewhere else (his laundry, of course, stays entirely at home). Your teen may have a part-time job, a driver's license, a girlfriend, and any number of sports and school activities. After all these years of training, he may be handy in the kitchen—too bad he's too busy to help!

Despite the attraction of the outside world, teenagers need their parents. Just as the toddler needed you to make it safe for him to walk on his own, your teen needs you to prepare him to walk right out your door. Don't be surprised if your teenager wants to do things his way—after all, he's had a mind of his own since he was a toddler!

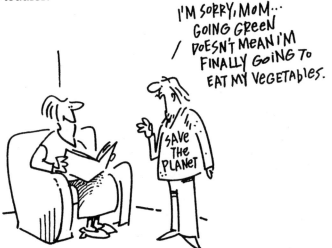

Your older teen may want to eat differently. He may move from being a fast-food fanatic to declining anything with a hint of fat. He may declare he's converting to vegetarianism, or complain that family foods affect his complexion. He may bring concoctions home from the gym and instruct you on his protein needs. What could be more interesting than living with a teenager?

Remind yourself that you have years of training. You're no longer that amateur cradling a tiny baby in your arms! Past experience will come in handy. Just as you let your toddler make some snack choices, or let your seven-year-old pack his lunch, give your older teen new responsibilities. Give him extra freedom, too—with age-appropriate limits. If he wants to go vegetarian while the rest of the family continues to eat meat, let him help with the purchase and preparation of his meat substitutes. Just as you didn't cater to a picky toddler, you needn't prepare separate meals for a demanding teenager. Give him suggestions for customizing family meals to meet his needs, but make sure to eat "his way" once in a while. Without compromising your preferences, show respect for his ideas.

Help your teen stay real. Become aware of outside influences that could compromise regular eating. Does the wrestling team encourage athletes to starve and dehydrate themselves to "make weight"? Does the running coach recommend meal patterns that leave kids hungry? How much of your teen's daily food comes from vending machines and fast-food outlets? Your older teenager may not want you to interfere, but open discussions at home will help him grapple with the issues.

Family mealtimes can keep teens grounded while letting their spirits soar. As a respite from the hectic, outside world, the dinner table can provide the right space for family members to slow down and eat mindfully, while staying connected to one another. Food fads will come and go, but the young adult who has mastered the "art of eating" will leave home with a good foundation for healthy living.

Because You Asked about How to Feed Your Family

Q: If I breastfeed, how will I be able to tell whether my baby's getting enough milk?

A: *Your baby is probably getting enough if he has at least six to eight wet diapers a day and regular bowel movements (don't worry about the color). It's important to weigh and measure him at the doctor's office or health clinic every few weeks to make sure he's growing steadily. Your baby may lose some weight during the first few days after birth, while your milk is coming in, so be sure to ask a nurse to jot down his weight on the day you leave the hospital. It may take a few days for him to get back to his birth-weight.*

Q: I want to be able to feed my baby when we go out, but I've heard it's unsafe to heat his bottle in a microwave. What should I do?

A: *Heating a bottle in a microwave oven can be dangerous. Glass bottles have been known to shatter and—regardless of the kind of bottle you use—microwave heating can cause "hot spots." Even if you test a few drops of milk on your wrist, there's a danger of your son getting a scalding gulp! Always remove the nipple before putting your baby's bottle in the microwave. Replace the nipple on the heated bottle, tipping the contents back and forth several times to distribute the warmth evenly. It won't hurt your infant to have a cold bottle (really, it won't!), but if you wish to take the chill off, there's a better way than microwaving. Ask your host to put the bottle in a bowl of warm water for a minute or two.*

Q: Robbie, our two-year-old, refuses to sit at the table to eat. To ensure he eats something, we let him take what he wants from the table so he can eat it as he plays in the kitchen.

A: *Your son may be getting some of the foods he needs, but he's not learning good eating habits. Robbie may also be paying more attention to his toys than his appetite! Tell him it's more fun to eat at the table, and let him choose where to sit. To signal the change, add a colorful table center or other decoration. During the meal, include him in the conversation without making him the center of attention. When he wants to get down, let him go, but don't let him take food with him. Tell him he's welcome to come back and eat some more. Stay low-key and relaxed—don't be critical if he fidgets or occasionally stands up (as long as he's in no danger of falling).*

Q: You don't advocate eating in the car, but we have a long commute twice a day with our preschoolers. The best way to keep them happy is to give them crackers and raisins while we're driving. Is it okay to let kids nibble on nutritious snacks?

A: *It's better for kids to eat in appropriate places where they can pay attention to eating—and you can respond quickly if someone starts to choke. An occasional car snack may be okay when there's another adult along, but snacking twice daily is liable to make kids want to eat every time they get into a car! Raisins and crackers aren't friendly to teeth—especially nibbled over time—and kids can choke easily on raisins. Raw veggies, cheese, and fruit are better snack foods—but if they're cut into small pieces, they may be messy to eat in the car. Make sure the kids have time to eat before the morning commute, and ask their caregiver to give them an afternoon snack to tide them over for the trip home. Look for ways to make the car ride fun for everyone, such as listening to taped stories or singing along to children's songs.*

Q: Mark, who's eight years old, hardly ever eats the lunch I pack him for school. He's ravenous after school, so he eats a huge snack. Then he's not very interested in dinner. Any suggestions?

A: *Going all day without food is hard on Mark. Because he's not eating, his blood-sugar levels will be especially low in the afternoon, making it difficult for him to concentrate on his studies. Speak to Mark about his reasons for not eating his lunch. Does he dislike the type of food you're packing? Is he eager to go out and play? Is he uncomfortable eating in front of other students? Contact his teacher to help clarify the situation. It's important to avoid forcing anything on Mark, but he may need lots of encouragement and support to turn this pattern around. Once he's agreed to eat at school, encourage him to pack his own lunch with your guidance.*

Q: Our 14-year-old daughter has started taking her dinner to her room. She likes to talk on the phone to friends or watch TV while she eats. How can we get her to join us in the dining room? She's gets testy when we insist.

A: *Tell her you'd like her company at dinner, and she can speak to her friends and watch TV at other times (avoid making these activities seem trivial!). What would make it more fun for her to eat with you? As a family, agree on the timing of the meal, the background music, and general topics of conversation. It's reasonable to ask her to sit with you for about 30 minutes before being excused.*

6

The Science of Eating

*Nature is generous. The earth
yields abundant wholesome food
to nourish body and soul.*

Visit a farmers' market at harvest time. You can create a small work of art just by filling your shopping basket! What you'll see is real food. If your child points at a vegetable and asks, "What's that, Mom?" you'll probably know the answer.

Imagine a time when that was the only way food was marketed. No in-your-face TV ads. No neon signs dotting the landscape. No flashy packages row on row at the store. Life's not that simple anymore. We watch TV. We follow neon signs. We heap our grocery carts with packages—though we'd be hard-pressed to help a child identify every ingredient!

Once in a while, close your eyes and visualize *your* favorite farmers' market. Fresh foods grown close to home and purchased in season are part of our heritage—a tradition shared by people from all over the globe. In many ways, market products still represent the best in quality, setting the standard for all our daily food choices.

Quality counts: The food you give your child today will have a lasting impact on her physical and mental development. Child nutrition experts Susan Roberts and Melvin Heyman, authors of *Feeding Your Child for Lifelong Health*, call it "metabolic programming." It means the food your child eats while her brain and other body tissues develop is important for life. As a parent, you have time-limited opportunities to ensure that your child gets optimal nutrition when she needs it most. The choices you make for your child today will program *her* choices in the future.

The previous chapter focused on *how* to eat. This chapter is about *what* to eat. It will guide you in providing your child with the best possible nourishment at each critical stage of growth and development. I'll begin with some nutrition basics for kids of all ages, and then take you through various stages, linking special topics to milestones in a child's life. Whatever your child's age, follow the chronological path—many topics introduced at one stage continue to be relevant at another.

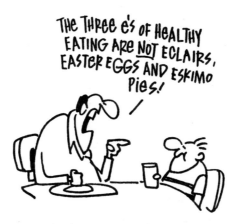

Real Food for Real Kids

Nothing we eat is absolutely perfect—or entirely bad. It's simplistic to claim some foods are good for us, while labeling others "junk." Well-meaning parents often do just that. They say, "Eat that kale, Joel. It will make you strong," and "Candy isn't good for you, Ashley. It'll rot your teeth and make you fat." Joel and Ashley love their parents and want to please them, but they know from experience that "bad" things often taste better than those considered "good." Playing "good food/bad food" causes needless conflict between parents and kids.

Classifying everything we eat as either good or bad doesn't help us make healthy choices, either. You'd probably consider carrots, oranges, and broccoli to be "good" foods. But if they were the only things your child ate, she wouldn't grow and thrive. To get all the nutrients her body needs, your child has to eat several different types of food. Worldwide, there are many eating styles, most of them based on three to six "food groups." The popular, practical "four food groups" include grain products, vegetables and fruit, milk and alternatives, and meat and alternatives. Today's "milk" and "meat" groups have changed to encompass vegetarian options. The "alternatives" for the milk group still include yogurt and cheese, but the group also embraces plant-based foods such as fortified soy drink, tofu made with calcium, leafy green vegetables, and almonds. Besides fish, poultry, and eggs, meat alternatives include plant-based foods such as dried beans, lentils, tofu, nuts, and seeds.

Each of the food groups has a distinctive pattern of nutrients and protective substances. Combine all four groups and they work together to build body cells and keep every system humming. There are dozens of nutrients, but it's not important that you know their names. I don't wander around the supermarket mumbling, "Magnesium, selenium, riboflavin ..." and you don't have to, either. Like me, you can simply fill your cart with a variety of foods from the basic groups.

I used to choose oranges for their vitamin C. Now I know that oranges also contain 150 different "phytochemicals" (plant chemicals) that can help keep my family healthy. What a bonus! It's clear that an orange has much more to offer than a vitamin C-fortified "fruit" drink. Vegetables and fruit come in many beautiful colors, which is Nature's way of encouraging us to eat a variety of them. In fact, the more different foods you choose, the more likely you'll provide your family with all the nutrients they need.

Whenever you make food choices, favor the basic, *less-processed* foods from each food group. Whole-grain breads and cereals will have more trace nutrients and fiber than the highly refined products. Fresh and frozen veggies and fruit offer more nutrients per bite than the ones with added fat or sugar. Empty-calorie foods, whose fat and sugar content overwhelm any other nutrients present, don't rate a place in a food group. But you needn't avoid them altogether. It won't harm most children to eat small amounts of these "extras" if nearly all the foods they eat are wholesome.

When you dine out, remember the same food-selection principles you follow at the grocery store. Nutrition often slips people's minds the moment they enter a restaurant. It's fine to "splurge" once in a while, but today people often eat out several times a week.

Choosing Champion Carbs

"Complex" carbohydrates are found in starchy foods such as whole-grain breads, cereals, pasta and rice, lentils, dried peas and beans, and some vegetables. These foods are minimally processed and nutrient-dense, and high in vitamins, minerals, and fiber.

"Simple" carbohydrates are found in regular soft drinks, candy, honey, jams, and sugary baked goods. Mainly comprising sugar, they're just "empty calories."

In between complex and simple carbohydrates come refined bread, cereal, pasta, and rice made from white processed grains. White bread and pasta made from enriched white flour are nutritious, but low in fiber and trace nutrients.

New research on the "glycemic index" is changing the way we look at starches and sugars. The glycemic index is a measure of how quickly the carbohydrate in a particular food is broken down to release sugar into the bloodstream. It measures how high your blood sugar rises after eating certain foods. High glycemic-index foods are digested quickly, causing a rapid increase (followed by a sudden drop) in blood sugar. This can leave you feeling hungry very soon after eating. Simple sugars usually have a high glycemic index, but so do some nutritious foods, such as potatoes. High-fiber foods—including most whole grains, beans, and vegetables (especially raw veggies)—tend to have a low glycemic index, giving them more "staying power." That's fine for older children and teens, but babies' and toddlers' digestive systems aren't proficient at breaking down fiber, which is why you'll see whole kernels of corn in their stools, and why you should limit their intake of high-fiber foods.

Calories can be confusing. They come from three sources: protein, carbohydrates, and fat. Because protein is needed for growth and repair of body tissues, we depend on carbohydrates and fat for most of our "food energy." Fat has twice as many calories as an equivalent amount of protein or carbohydrate, so a small serving of a high-fat food will pack as many calories as a larger serving of food high in carbs or protein. Studies show that North Americans have cut back on fat, but we're making up for it by eating more carbohydrates—and more calories—than ever!

Are foods high in fats and carbohydrates always "fattening"? Some kids worry so much about fattening food they're embarrassed to be seen buying a chocolate bar. Yet we know people can eat chocolate without getting fat. We also know some people struggle with their weight no matter what they eat. Kids put on extra weight if they eat more than they need for growth and activity.

That can happen regardless of where the calories come from. A child can gain extra weight by eating or drinking too much of anything, including healthy foods.

Choosing First-Rate Fats

In moderate amounts, fat is as important to health as any other nutrient, but some types of fat are healthier than others. Fats are named according to their chemical make-up. "Unsaturated" fats, found in olive and canola oils and fish, are considered healthier than the "saturated" fats found in most meat, dairy products, and coconut oil. The *least* healthy choice is "trans" fat, formed when liquid oils are made solid by a process called hydrogenation. Why the concern? Saturated and trans fats can raise blood levels of LDL (low-density lipoprotein) or "bad" cholesterol. Cholesterol is a natural substance our bodies produce. It's a problem only if we have too much of the "bad" type coursing through our arteries, raising the risk of heart disease. Get your fat from foods that contain unsaturated fats such as fish, nuts, seeds, avocado, non-hydrogenated margarines, and olive, canola, and fish oils. They provide essential fatty acids that will enable you to absorb and use the fat-soluble vitamins: A, D, E, and K.

Throughout this book, I emphasize the importance of variety. Like all good rules, this one has an exception. People who eat a lot of different foods *high in fat and sugar* tend to gain extra weight. Perhaps their mouths still want more when their stomachs tell them they've eaten enough! Many people get used to eating about the same volume at meals and snacks, regardless of how filling the individual foods are. When that happens, they can't depend on their appetites to tell them that a small amount of a high-calorie food goes a long way. When you think "variety" in your meal planning, don't extend the concept to foods high in fat and sugar—with "extras," your child is likely to want to try a little of everything.

You may wonder how much your child should eat at each stage. The table on page 142 provides ballpark figures—but that's all they are. Each child is unique. Children of the same age are often different sizes, so it stands to reason that they'd have different calorie needs. Because it's difficult to figure out just how much food your child needs, it's best to let her follow her appetite. Watch for balance in the amounts she eats from each food group. There should be two or three times as many servings from the grains group and vegetables group as from the milk and meat groups. And—this is important—whatever a child's stage of development, "extras" shouldn't overshadow the basics. I've seen this happen when a youngster takes two spoons of veggies, a bite or two of meat, and then completes her "mini-meal" with an adult-size piece of cake!

Just as no food can guarantee good health on its own, no food is so bad that it will undermine a child's well-being if eaten in moderation. I always remind myself that good health doesn't depend on food alone. Exercise, rest, proper hygiene, and plenty of love are absolutely essential. Let's go back to Joel and Ashley—the kids whose parents gave them "good food/bad food" advice. If Joel eats many different wholesome foods and leads an active life, he'll probably grow up strong—whether or not he eats kale. And if Ashley eats well, plays hard, and takes care of her teeth, a little candy shouldn't harm her!

The Infant – Safe and Sound

Babies are small and vulnerable. Feeding them has as much to do with protecting them from harm as with good nutrition. Colostrum, the first substance moms' breasts secrete, is rich in antibodies that help protect a baby from infections and allergies before her own immune system kicks in. If a mom, dad, or sibling has an allergy to any food, it's wise to breastfeed a baby for at least six months before offering her *any* other food or drink. (A vitamin D supplement *may* be the exception. Because babies in northern countries often have limited exposure to sunshine, a pediatric vitamin D supplement is recommended for some breastfed infants. Ask your doctor or public health nurse to advise you.)

A child whose family history makes her susceptible to allergies is more likely to become allergic to foods such as cow's milk or soy products if she's given them early in infancy. That's because an immature digestive system may not fully break down the protein from cow's milk or soy, and absorption of these protein fragments can trigger an allergic response. If your child is at risk, wait until she's 12 months old before introducing cow's milk, shellfish, egg yolks, soy, or chopped peanuts or nuts. Egg whites—whether raw or cooked—can cause a reaction even in babies who *aren't* particularly susceptible to allergies, so wait until she's one before offering whole eggs.

Recognizing Food Sensitivities

A true food allergy—in which the body makes antibodies in response to a specific food protein—doesn't happen as often as you may think. Studies show that five to eight percent of children under the age of three develop a food allergy. Within the total population, however, just one to two percent are allergic to food. Most food allergies are to cow's milk, eggs, soybeans, wheat, fish, shellfish, peanuts, and nuts. Children often outgrow allergies to milk, eggs, soy, and wheat by the time they're five, while peanut, nut, fish, and shellfish allergies often continue for decades or more.

A child may be sensitive to a food without being allergic to it. Lactose intolerance is a digestive problem that occurs when a person is low in "lactase," the enzyme that breaks down milk sugar. Someone with lactose intolerance may have enough lactase to eat some types of yogurt and cheese, and even drink small amounts of milk without discomfort. An intestinal infection can cause a temporary intolerance to lactose in babies. If your baby's formula makes her gassy and uncomfortable after an illness, ask your doctor to recommend a lactose-free formula until her digestive system recovers. Don't restrict lactose longer than necessary—it's a natural ingredient in human and animal milk that aids calcium absorption and brain development.

If your baby screams with frequent tummy aches, develops a rash, or has a constantly running nose, ask your doctor's advice. The cramps and fussiness we call "colic" are sometimes related to food. A bottle-fed baby may become allergic to her formula, or a breastfed baby may become sensitive to something her mom eats. Don't make your own diagnosis—I wouldn't! There's no sense putting unnecessary restrictions on what you or your baby has to eat. Even more important, your baby's signs of distress could indicate a serious health problem. Because some intestinal disorders are rare, they're often misdiagnosed as an allergy or routine fussiness.

Whether or not you breastfeed your baby, you may want to give her an infant formula at some point, either as a supplement or a replacement for your milk when you stop breastfeeding. Choose a breast-milk substitute with care, seeking advice from a doctor or dietitian if the formula doesn't seem to agree with your baby. It'll be easier on your baby if you can avoid making needless changes. For babies less than one year of age, select an iron-fortified infant formula based on cow's milk ("follow on" formulas developed for babies over six months are unnecessary). While cow's milk itself isn't recommended for babies under one, formulas *based* on cow's milk come closest to approximating the composition of breast milk. Some formula companies try to mimic breast milk by adding special fats and other ingredients believed to enhance infant development. Despite these new advances, no manufacturer has yet duplicated mother's milk. (Avoid feeding your baby homemade evaporated cow's or goat's milk formula. These formulas are low in iron and essential fatty acids, and their high concentration of protein and minerals can put a strain on a baby's kidneys.)

Although they remain an option for families that want to avoid animal-based products, soy-based formulas have fallen out of favor with some medical experts. One drawback is the possible effect of soy's natural estrogen content. Plant estrogens in soy are beneficial for menopausal women, but their effects on babies are unknown. Soy also lacks lactose. In the past, soy formula was recommended for babies allergic to cow's milk, but we now know that infants with milk allergies may develop a cross sensitivity to soy.

Drinks—sometimes called "milks"—made from soy, rice, almond, or any other type of plant *do not meet an infant's needs*, regardless of whether they're fortified with added nutrients. Soy drinks or "milks" are distinctly different from soy-based infant formulas and are not suitable for children under two. If you give your baby soy formula, keep her on it until age two, unless she's getting whole cow's milk after her first birthday.

If your baby's allergic to milk, the best choice may be a special formula in which the cow's milk protein has been broken down for easy digestion. Ask a dietitian or public health nurse for a specific recommendation.

Infant formula comes ready to use, or as a liquid concentrate or powder. When mixing it, follow package directions exactly, under scrupulously clean conditions. For babies less than four months, water used for mixing formula must be boiled for two minutes, then cooled. Formula that's too concentrated, too dilute, or unhygienic can be harmful to babies.

The Older Baby - Brain Food First!

If men are from Mars and women are from Venus, babies must be from an entirely different planet! Since their brains are still under construction, babies' nutritional needs are different from those of older kids and adults. After birth, a child experiences rapid brain growth that continues until about age three. Mother's milk is ideally suited to help this process—half its calories come from fat, a nutrient needed in generous amounts for brain and spinal cord development. (Studies show breastfed babies often score higher on intelligence tests than formula-fed babies.)

With past generations, no one worried about limiting fat in childhood, so "brain food" for babies wasn't an issue. Babies were often breastfed for two years or longer, ensuring a good supply of essential fatty acids. With today's concerns about heart disease and excess weight, however, most families use reduced-fat milk—and are eager to give it to their babies, too.

Pediatric and dietetic associations recommend weaning babies to whole cow's milk (3.5% milk fat) after at least one year on breast milk or infant formula. After age two, a child can be given 2% milk as a matter of convenience, but it's not necessary to switch. Children older than two who eat a wide variety of wholesome foods can gradually move from 2% to 1% to skim milk. Health authorities in the U.S. recommend following this sequence in early childhood, so that by the time a child is a preschooler, she's drinking skim milk. Some Canadian guidelines suggest kids should reach their full height before switching to skim milk.

This wide disparity in American and Canadian guidelines demonstrates just how controversial nutrition can be! I gave skim milk to my daughters when they were preteens. Because they found it thirst quenching, they drank more—something I wanted to encourage. Our family continued to eat cheese and other wholesome foods that contain fat. Real foods that are higher in fat shouldn't be restricted to the same extent as fatty snack foods.

Speaking of real food, it's time! In the previous chapter, I explained why babies are ready for solid food at four to six months, and how to introduce your little one to this new eating experience. Now I'll focus on specific foods appropriate for babies. Whether your child eagerly licks her lips, or shows little interest in the strange stuff on the spoon, this is a big step. When choosing your baby's first foods, there are several important things to consider: her readiness to eat and digest solids, her nutrient needs, and food safety.

Iron-fortified infant cereals meet all of a baby's needs for a first food. After about six months, the iron stores babies are born with begin to dwindle. Since breast milk is low in iron, breastfed babies in particular need a good source when they're ready for solid food. Like fat, iron is critically important for the development of the central nervous system. A lack of iron not only affects the brain's growth—it can undermine a child's capacity to learn. Babies who experience even a mild iron deficiency may suffer permanent mental and motor impairments.

Offer single-grain cereals first, starting with iron-fortified rice cereal, followed by barley and oat cereals. This sequence puts foods less likely to cause an adverse reaction first. If you introduce one food at a time (with four to seven days between new selections), it'll be easier to identify the offending food if your baby has an allergic reaction. Two or three weeks after introducing cereal, start giving her plain well-mashed vegetables, one at a time. Because babies prefer the sweet taste of fruit, it's better to offer vegetables first.

Nutritionists no longer recommend *puréed* vegetables and fruit—they lack texture. Instead, offer your baby soft, *mashed* veggies and fruit. It's quite convenient to simply mash and mince the food you've cooked for the family—as long as you haven't added salt or sugar. If you use canned vegetables and fruit, choose those without added sugar, salt, or other additives. Root vegetables such as carrots may be too high in nitrates for babies under six months—another reason not to rush solids.

You may wish to freeze batches of mashed veggies in ice-cube trays, before transferring the chunks to freezer bags. That's a real time-saver if you process baby food in a blender: Small portions thaw fast and help you minimize waste (leftovers must be thrown out). When your baby's ready for meat, poultry, or fish, cook it, then chop it very finely, moistening with a little water.

Some babies love solid food—and there's no stopping them. They cheerfully down their cereal, veggies, and fruit, and their equally cheerful parents proceed to offer them meat, fish, poultry, beans, tofu—you name it! Other babies aren't so keen. With time, all babies learn to eat solid food. Watch for any sign of enthusiasm and capitalize on it. Does "Miss Picky" pick up tiny pieces of food from her high-chair tray? Offer her finger foods—peeled soft fruit, cooked vegetable chunks, cooked pasta, toast, crackers, "oat ring" cereal, and pieces of soft cheese. Follow your baby's lead.

Most commercial baby foods don't offer the texture babies need to ease them into eating regular family food. Commercial foods also tend to be more expensive than homemade, although there may be times when their convenience makes them worth the cost. Many baby-food manufacturers now avoid the use of additives. If you buy commercial baby foods, choose single-food items. Mixed dinners are not good value—and it's hard to estimate how much of each ingredient a baby eats. Beware of regular products such as apple juice sold in baby-sized jars at several times the price of regular juice.

Babies don't need juice. That may surprise you, but they really don't! Do give your baby fruit, which contains all the nutrients found in juice, and more. Even diluted juice is hard on babies' tender new teeth, especially if it's sucked from a bottle. A "sip cup," equipped with a spout on the lid, can also contribute to tooth decay if a baby carries it around, sipping frequently. If you want to give your baby a sip cup, limit its use to meal and snack times except when it's filled with water.

Anything sweet can be hard on your baby's teeth, especially if it's also sticky. Even healthy foods such as dried apricots, peaches, and raisins can cause decay. Baby teeth are important. If they become decayed, the infection can affect a child's permanent teeth, which erupt later. Some preschoolers endure multiple tooth extractions because their parents allowed them to nibble on dried fruit from babyhood, or to suck on a pacifier dipped in honey.

Safety continues to be a priority for the older baby. Honey—whether pasteurized or not—shouldn't be given to babies before their first birthday because it may contain spores that cause infant botulism. And never pop a raw egg into a salad dressing or blender drink. The slight chance of bacterial contamination makes raw eggs unsuitable for young children, pregnant women, and people with weakened immune systems.

Chop all foods finely to lessen your baby's risk of choking, and never leave babies and young children to eat or drink unattended. Spread peanut butter thinly on bread or crackers, rather than offering it alone or on a spoon.

The Toddler - Sweetheart with a Sweet Tooth

Toddlers are happy snackers. Snacks satisfy their small appetites, short attention span, and newfound "pester power." Some snacks are so tasty that toddlers beg for more, blunting their appetite for the next meal. It's easy to see how a frustrating cycle can develop. Kids who are too full from snacks don't want to eat their vegetables or try new foods. At meals, they nibble and fidget—then fuel up again with the next snack.

Think "balance" with your toddler. Balance in the feeding relationship between you and your child. Balance among the four food groups—even at snack time! Balance between high-nutrient foods and low-nutrient extras at meals and snacks. And balance between solids and liquids.

When a parent calls me to say her toddler doesn't eat, I usually discover the child does a great deal of drinking. Many a toddler favors a liquid diet, especially when the drinks are sweet. Even 100 percent fruit juice is high in sugar. Kids who fill up on juice can miss out on important nutrients from other foods. Too much fruit juice, especially apple juice, has also been linked with chronic diarrhea in young children. If your child has diarrhea, it's not a good idea to give her apple juice—something that was commonly recommended in the past.

It's easy for kids to drink too much juice, partly because they like the sweet taste. But there's also another reason: Because calories from drinks may not curb the appetite as much as calories from solid food, a child may just keep on drinking, unaware that she's had enough. Be sure to let your toddler quench her thirst with water whenever she wants to, but limit juice to about one-half cup (125 mL) a day, preferably adding water to double the volume. Limit milk intake to two to three cups (500 to 750 mL) a day.

Too much sweet food can throw a toddler's diet off balance, too. We taste food *milliseconds* after it touches our tongues. Sugar almost instantly stimulates the release of the feel-good brain chemicals called endorphins. Offer sweet treats—even delicious home-baked ones—less often and in smaller quantities than basic foods. Toddlers with tiny appetites don't have as much "room" for extras as children who eat larger amounts of wholesome foods.

Parents often ask me for snack recipes for their toddlers. Rather than providing special "snack" foods, offer toddlers real food at snack time—plain fruits and vegetables and low-sugar cereals and muffins—to complement what they eat at mealtime. Reserve sweets for occasional desserts after meals, when a child's appetite is already partly satisfied.

A toddler needs plenty of guidance as she wobbles into our world! This is an important time for parents, grandparents, friends, and neighbors to stick together, offering a little person the highest quality foods. Don't ban grandma's cookies or fret over birthday parties, but stay "in charge" when it comes to food selection. Eating healthy foods is fun, especially when pancakes look like Mickey Mouse and sandwiches are cut into triangles and squares. If Lucy eats too much candy at a neighbor's house today, don't try to restrict her eating tomorrow. That will only contribute to a feast-and-fast mentality that can upset her body's natural ability to regulate her eating. Each day, make a fresh start.

The Preschooler – The Consumer's Apprentice

Most preschoolers have discovered that food isn't just about nourishment, or even about feeling good. Now it has entertainment value! Cereal can look and taste like candy. Fruit can be flattened, rolled, and packaged into tidy little servings. Yogurt comes in cute tubs and snazzy tubes. Special kids' meals are packaged in cool boxes, with collectible toys inside! Ain't life grand!

If you close your eyes, maybe you can still visualize the scene at the farmers' market! Try hard—your preschooler needs you to maintain that perspective. The occasional fast-food meal or packaged snack won't hurt, if healthy basics remain the mainstay of your little one's regular eating pattern. Go ahead and give your preschooler choices—between blueberries and a banana, or between muffins made with raisins or apples. Have fun with real food. Put a vegetable for tonight's dinner in a big paper bag and let your preschooler guess what's inside. When she "solves the mystery," give her a taste of the veggie before you cook it. When she quotes TV ads, ask her to help you "advertise" the wonderful foods you plan to make for dinner by coloring pictures to hang in the kitchen. Give her some bean seeds to plant so she can watch them grow. A child with a garden gains a whole new perspective on veggies!

Preschoolers seem to vacillate between periods of eager eating and times when real food holds little appeal. The child who used to hang around the kitchen asking for handouts suddenly has to be called to dinner. Help her balance her choices by offering her wholesome foods she already enjoys along with new foods she's still learning to like. This is a stage when nutrient supplements can help fill the gaps left by finicky eating. Surveys show that many preschoolers don't get all the nutrients they require even when they eat enough calories. If your child doesn't seem to be eating enough from all four food groups, ask a pharmacist or dietitian to help you choose a multivitamin and mineral pill formulated especially for children. But keep in mind that no pill can provide the full health protection of natural food.

Vitamin pills can seem like a "treat" to kids. Many look like candy and taste like it, too—but they're not innocuous. Handle supplements as if they were medicine, keeping them out of children's reach and doling them out, usually no more than one a day. Too much of some vitamins and minerals can cause illness—a situation that can easily happen if *both* parents give her a vitamin pill each day. There's only a threefold difference between the amount of vitamin D a child requires, and the amount that can disturb bone development! Zinc, iron, and vitamin A are also toxic in large doses. And even vitamin C—so casually scarfed down by young and old—can upset the balance of other essential nutrients if you take too much.

"Nutraceuticals"—part food, part supplement—also target little consumers who'd rather pop a pill than eat their veggies. Of course, there's no magic way to squeeze the essence of several vegetables into one tiny tablet, although many busy parents wish it were possible! "Functional foods" are designed to provide "added" health benefits beyond basic nutrition. Some manufacturers spike foods and drinks with one or two nutrients that tend to be lacking in some kids' diets—and market them in eye-catching packages. Unfortunately, a child who isn't getting enough calcium, for example, probably isn't getting enough of the other nutrients she needs, either. A brightly colored, sugary drink with added calcium won't do much to balance her diet.

Artificial sweeteners and fat substitutes have also found their way into foods popular with kids. The common sweetener aspartame is made from two naturally occurring amino acids. The amount of aspartame in one diet soda probably won't harm a child, but some kids down several artificially flavored drinks and snack foods daily. Each one takes the place of another beverage or food—one that could give a child the nutrients she needs. Young kids don't need fat substitutes, either. Some fat replacements cause gas and sudden diarrhea, and reduce the absorption of fat-soluble vitamins. When in doubt about a food choice, stay real! As inventive as they are, food technologists are hard-pressed to improve on Nature.

The Primary School Child - Six Going on Sixteen

The primary school child has more discretion over what she eats than ever before in her short life! When she goes "trick or treating" or attends a birthday party, she brings home her own private stash. She has spending power. She influences family food choices. She also begins to eat more meals away from home — and with each passing year, her teachers pay less attention to her lunch box.

A recent study showed one in five kids goes to school on an empty stomach. While poverty can be a factor, many kids — even little ones — skip breakfast because they're weight-conscious. Children who skip meals or restrict themselves to too few foods often don't do well at school, lacking the energy and attention span needed for active learning.

Balanced breakfasts and nourishing lunches can help a child learn more and have more fun playing. Anything that's quick, easy, and tasty is right for breakfast — even leftover pizza with a glass of milk and a juicy orange. Try to include selections from three or four food groups at every meal. Studies show that few children come close to eating the recommended amounts of vegetables and fruit. Maybe they'd do better if they chose real food for snacks. Many kids don't eat enough meat or alternatives, either. What *do* kids eat? Grains seem to be the only food group we can usually count on children eating in sufficient amounts.

Today's kids drink less milk than ever before. Parents are drinking less milk, too — ostensibly to reduce their fat intake. Why do people cut back on milk rather than switch to 1% or skim? Blame it on our collective sweet tooth, or the marketing power of the soft drink industry. Today, North Americans spend more on soft drinks, juices, and fruit-flavored drinks than on milk. Colas are among the most popular drinks in the entire world!

Earlier, I claimed no food was indispensable, but milk is such an important source of calcium and vitamin D that it deserves special mention. You may think of osteoporosis as an adult disease because it strikes people in midlife, but doctors are beginning to refer to it as a pediatric disease. The reason? While calcium continues to be important throughout life for bones' maintenance and repair, its effect on bone density is particularly important in childhood. *Kids reach their peak bone mass at the end of adolescence.* Parents of kids who don't drink much milk often tell me their kids are healthy. But high bone density isn't obvious to the naked eye—it can't even be seen on ordinary X-rays. Your child can appear to be healthy while missing a time-limited opportunity to build strong bones for life.

The child who drinks mostly juice and soda in the first grade isn't going to switch to milk in her teens! Ensure that your child's calcium intake isn't interrupted during her early school years. Children can get calcium from milk substitutes such as tofu and leafy greens, but they may not eat these foods every day or in sufficient quantities. Soy drinks can substitute for milk when children are two or older, as long as the drinks are fortified with calcium and vitamin D. If you suspect your child is not getting enough milk or suitable alternatives, discuss her eating habits with a dietitian or pediatrician.

The effect of eating on child behavior has sparked much interest in the past 20 years, particularly since the publication in the late 1970s of Dr. Ben Feingold's *Why Your Child Is Hyperactive.* Feingold suggested a direct cause and effect between hyperactivity and kids' diets, especially when artificial colors and flavors and "salicylates"—compounds found in some additives and natural foods—are present. What *really* caught the collective imagination was the idea that sugary "junk" foods and candy might make kids "hyperactive." Parents and teachers alike opined that even mild-mannered kids bounced off the walls under the influence of sugar.

Don't believe all the "sweet talk" you hear. Scientific studies don't support the sugar and hyperactivity theory. In fact, like all carbohydrates, sugar can have a mild sedative effect since it tends to boost the levels of serotonin—a brain chemical that makes people drowsy. Much of the hype about sugar is due to guilt by association. Kids get excited at parties and special events, sometimes "losing" it due to simple exhaustion. Still, when eating is unbalanced—with more empty-calorie items than health-building foods—kids can't be expected to behave well, especially if their snacks include a hit of caffeine. Children's blood-sugar levels are steadier when they eat balanced meals. When you look for a connection between food and behavior, it's important to distinguish between healthy kids who sometimes eat poorly, and children who have a behavioral ailment such as attention deficit disorder, which may or may not be related to what they eat.

Recognizing ADHD

We hear a lot about attention deficit/hyperactivity disorder (ADHD) these days, partly because of better detection and treatment. A child with ADHD (or ADD, as it's sometimes called) "reacts" rather than "responds" to situations. He's not being willful or stubborn—he has a brain-wiring problem beyond his control.

It takes a skilled professional with expertise in this area to make a diagnosis: Not every impulsive or hyperactive child actually has this disorder. The American Academy of Pediatrics says clues that a child may have ADD include at least a six-month history of troubled relationships at home and at school, academic underachievement, and behavioral problems present in two or more of his usual settings. The observations of parents, caregivers, classroom teachers, or other school professionals should all be considered, as should the possibility of coexisting conditions such as learning and language problems, aggression, disruptive behavior, depression, or anxiety.

The Canadian Pediatric Society (CPS) suggests boredom, depression, family issues, physical illness, undiagnosed sight or hearing problems, inappropriate expectations, a mismatch between teacher and child, or teacher incompetence could all contribute to a child's inattention and impulsivity.

The CPS recommends that physicians consider if such problems are present before making a diagnosis. The disorder affects an estimated four to 12 percent of school-aged youngsters—generally twice as many boys as girls. Children with ADHD benefit from regular, healthy meals and snacks, and often from medication. If you suspect that your child has ADHD or any other behavioral problem, contact the doctor, nurse, or counselor most familiar with your child and with this disorder.

Don't overlook the possibility of food sensitivities that may affect your child's behavior. Some young patients do show improved behavior and some sleep better after several weeks on a test diet that excludes substances such as artificial colors, flavors, or monosodium glutamate (MSG). If your child shows signs of having a behavioral problem, ask your doctor to refer you to a dietitian or allergist to check for possible food sensitivities.

The Preteen – Power Child

Your preteen may seem independent, but she needs you as much as ever—both as a role model and a staunch supporter. A recent study of 2,000 Canadian kids linked "feeling cared for" with a variety of healthy habits. Kids from nine to 12 who said they felt cared for, liked themselves, and considered their bodies "just right" were more likely to eat breakfast, a recess snack, and lunch. They were also more likely to be physically active at school, and less likely to be on a diet. Kids whose parents ate breakfast were almost twice as likely to eat breakfast themselves as kids whose parents skipped that first meal of the day.

The preteen has plenty of power to think and act. Harness that budding intellect and physical stamina to household decisions and tasks! Encourage your preteen to suggest recipes and express her creativity in the kitchen. When shortcuts are important, favor "speed scratch cooking" over fast-food takeouts. Prewashed veggies, bottled marinades, and fast-cooking pastas such as ravioli and tortellini can help you and your child put healthy meals on the table in minutes. For healthy snacks, buy fruit by the case when the price is right, and let your child and her friends help themselves to reasonable amounts. Kids this age need ready access to plenty of healthy food.

This is the time to delight in the present with your liberal-minded offspring, while paving the way for the teen years ahead. Talk about food-related issues as they come up in movies, TV shows, or the daily paper. Here's the tricky part: Try to avoid being judgmental. Instead of saying, "That silly girl ate only lettuce for dinner!" try "What do you think of the way that girl was eating?" Instead of, "Isn't it crazy that boys your age waste money on useless pills?" try "What do you think of young guys taking supplements to build their muscles?" You don't have to have all the answers—questions make better conversation starters!

Your preteen may need a reminder about the effect of food on dental health. Even very young children have heard the message that sugar isn't good for teeth, but your preteen may not know that starchy foods like potato chips break down to form sugars. Munching on chips all evening is harder on teeth than polishing off a candy bar in one minute flat! Snacking on raw vegetables can help clean the teeth as well as keeping gums and jaw bones healthy. Raw fruit also makes a good snack—a drink of water helps wash away any residue of the fruit's natural sugar. Keep a chilled selection of sliced peeled veggies and fruits on hand for snack attacks. Regular soft drinks aren't good for teeth—but neither are diet colas. The acid in soft drinks, citrus fruits, and pickles can erode tooth enamel.

The Younger Teen – Food and Mood

Your younger teen's focus is her body. She'll be pleased that you share her chief interest! Your challenge will be to help her take care of that wonderful body without developing an unhealthy obsession about it. Puberty's hormonal changes produce mood swings in girls. One minute, she's laughing hysterically on the phone. The next, she's slouched in her room with nothing good to say to anyone. Tears come more easily than ever. This can be a bewildering stage. One mother described her daughter's 13th year as 12 solid months of PMS! Regular eating can steady blood-sugar levels—and everyone's nerves! *What* your child eats makes a difference, too.

A snack of candy and a soft drink has two strikes against it. Its high sugar content will cause blood-sugar levels to rise sharply, then fall just as fast. The soft drink's caffeine will enhance the "sugar high." Snacks that combine complex carbohydrates with protein will help keep your child on an even keel. She could add a slice of cheese to a high-fiber muffin, or top whole-grain cereal with milk. The carbohydrates and protein will work together to boost the levels of "serotonin" in her brain, helping her feel relaxed. The fat and fiber in these snacks slows their digestion, preventing spikes and sudden drops in blood-sugar levels.

Since the female cycle is intimately related to metabolism, your daughter may crave sweet, fatty foods at certain times of the month. That may be one of the ways Nature helps a girl develop a womanly body. Teach your daughter to respect her body's signals. It often feels better—physically *and* psychologically—to eat a small piece of chocolate with a glass of skim milk, than to eat a large piece, or none at all. Boys often crave high-protein foods during their adolescent growth spurt, perhaps because they're building muscle mass.

Sports nutrition is a hot topic at junior high schools. It's relevant to young teens, regardless of their activity level, and it's helpful if parents understand the connections between food and sport. Your child will talk about her calorie needs for sports, and wonder about special sports bars and drinks. Boys tend to focus on what they should eat to build big muscles. All athletes need plenty of fluids to stay well hydrated. They also face the challenge of coordinating their eating and drinking with their practices and games. Sports can help your teenager feel good about herself, so do what you can to support her training schedule. This may mean some changes to the grocery list and family meal times.

Your teen's energy needs are high while she's growing, and extra activity will boost them higher still. This is not the time to go on a diet, but many weight-conscious teens try to train hard on minuscule servings. Encourage your teenager to follow her appetite, choosing foods from all four food groups. "Energy" bars can be convenient snacks, though they aren't necessary. Does working out make your teen hungrier? Congratulate her! That's a sign that her body knows what it needs. Too many girls are afraid of hunger, and try to ignore it. That only leads to a frustrating cycle of eating too little, then eating too much.

Girls *and* boys can meet most of their nutrient needs with ordinary, nourishing food, with the possible exception of iron. Young athletes need extra iron to make up for the demands of growth and muscle wear and tear. Girls lose additional iron through menstruation. Boys may need extra for bodybuilding. Teens low in iron tire easily. Your doctor can perform a simple blood test to see if your child needs an iron supplement.

Boys entering their growth spurt have high protein needs, particularly if they're working out. Years ago, boys used to ask me if they should eat more steak; today, they ask about protein powders. It's not unreasonable for boys to want to stock up on raw materials for the bulging biceps they covet. Your son may be hungry enough to eat more of everything (with some kids, that's an understatement!). He should be able to meet his protein needs by eating foods from the milk and meat groups at every meal. A well-nourished kid will be able to build muscle without eating huge portions of meat or taking protein supplements. If your son insists he needs extra protein, it won't hurt to pick up some skim milk powder for fortifying his blender drinks and cereals. To build and repair muscle, his body will take what it needs from the protein in his food. Amino acid supplements can disturb protein balance, so I always advise teen bodybuilders to avoid taking them. Too much protein or amino acids can also stress the kidneys and liver and contribute to dehydration.

Water is essential for every system of the body. All teenagers need plenty of fluids, and those who are developing extra muscle through sport need even more. Not drinking enough fluids can make a kid tired and cranky. In extreme cases, it can be lethal. Because they sweat less and their core temperatures rise faster, kids and teens are much more likely than adults to become overheated. Fruit juices and sports drinks can help your teen stay refreshed, but during intense activity, she may feel better drinking plain water. Sugar in fruit juice and sports drinks temporarily draws extra fluids into the stomach. This can produce a bloated feeling that's uncomfortable during a game or run. Still, if kids prefer flavored drinks during sports, let them have them. The important thing is to drink enough. Encourage your teen to drink until she doesn't feel thirsty, and then suggest she drink an additional glass.

In sports, as in life, timing is everything! A teen playing a sport doesn't want to be hungry when she starts the game, nor does she want to be digesting her last meal. The best solution is small frequent meals and snacks. Whether swimming, running, or playing a team sport, it's best to eat one to three hours before an activity, choosing easily digested, light meals. Your teen might have a package of instant oatmeal mixed with a half-cup of skim milk or soy drink, for example. After the game, a bean burrito with salsa and a glass of orange juice may go down well. When she's running late, suggest tuna and crackers, drinkable fruit-flavored yogurt, or a fruit smoothie made with milk. When your teen snacks with friends, suggest raw veggies with low-fat dip or unbuttered popcorn seasoned with grated Parmesan cheese.

The Older Teenager – Experimental Journey

Your older teenager lives in a world where people are judged by what they eat. Women who eat small portions are often considered more feminine and attractive than hearty eaters. In one study, subjects watched videos of the same average-size woman eating four different meals. When she ate a small salad, they considered her more attractive than when she bit into a big meatball sandwich! No wonder many girls have "dietary schizophrenia," swinging between tiny meals and big, high-calorie snacks. This is a good time to help girls and boys alike (and maybe Mom and Dad!) learn about reasonable serving sizes. A large muffin is equal to at least two standard servings of grains. A one-liter soft drink is about six times the size of one standard serving of fruit juice. A "big eat" chocolate bar is about 75 percent larger than a regular bar.

As a parent, this is also a good time to reflect on your attitudes toward *your* body weight and eating habits. You and your teen may share a similar body build, but whether you do or not, talk candidly about how your own body image has changed over the years. I know one mother who always felt "fat" as a teenager, and yet when her daughters tried on old clothes from her teen years, they fit! She couldn't believe she'd been the same size as her lovely teenagers.

Weight consciousness and environmental awareness have fueled a new interest in vegetarianism among teens. It's healthy to eat vegetarian if wholesome foods from all the food groups are part of the plan. But too many teens simply ignore the meat at family meals, and try to live on salads and bread. Some kids use vegetarianism as an excuse to skip family meals altogether. One anxious mom called me to ask what to feed a "vegetarian" daughter who didn't like vegetables! Studies show teen vegetarians often don't get enough energy, protein, calcium, iron, and zinc. Talk to your teenager about the type of vegetarianism she wants to embrace, and show her how to get the nutrients she needs. If you have a daughter, let her know her nutritional health as a teenager will affect her later ability to become a mom.

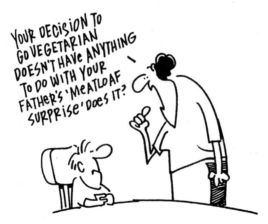

Some vegetarians eat everything except red meat. Others avoid animal flesh, but eat eggs and dairy products. "Vegans" avoid all animal-based products. If your teen doesn't want to eat dairy products, she'll need tofu made with calcium, fortified soy drinks, almonds and sesame seeds, and generous servings of leafy green vegetables. She'll also need vitamin B_{12} (available in supplements and some types of nutritional yeast) and vitamin D, found in vitamin supplements and some margarines (check the labels).

Red meat, by the way, isn't the villain your teen may imagine it to be. Small servings of lean cuts—baked, broiled, or occasionally barbecued—can make a nutrient-rich contribution to a balanced meal. Recent studies indicate fat from beef and dairy products may also help prevent breast cancer. Cows and other ruminants have a special kind of fat in their meat and milk that's been shown to kill cancer cells. Scientists say it's most important to get this particular essential fatty acid during the teen years, when girls' breasts are still developing.

Teenagers often limit their food choices because they're worried about their complexions. Roughly half of all teen visits to the doctor concern skin problems. Acne is a normal part of life for many teens, and while diet is often blamed, carefully controlled studies show no foods are consistently linked to the appearance or severity of acne. Eating a balanced diet with adequate amounts of vitamin A from dairy products and vegetables, and zinc from meat, fish, and poultry may improve your teen's complexion somewhat. There are several acne medications that are so high in vitamin A that they can cause birth defects if girls who use them get pregnant. Your daughter's doctor may routinely prescribe contraceptive pills along with these medications, regardless of whether your daughter is sexually active.

As you explore your teen's food-related interests and anxieties, try to keep an open mind and help her investigate new ideas. Watch for tips and recipes in her magazines, as well as yours. This is the time to help your teen refine the eating habits she'll take with her when she heads off into that wide world beyond the security of home.

Because You Asked What to Feed Your Family

Q: My husband and I are vegans, and the proud parents of a baby girl. Right now I'm breastfeeding her, but soon she'll be eating solid food. We want to raise our daughter on plant foods, but we don't want her to miss out on any important nutrients.

A: *The food your baby eats for the first three years must be high in fat, calcium, and iron—nutrients commonly found in animal-based foods. Some vegan parents find it easier to meet their children's nutrient needs if they offer them milk products, particularly during the preschool years. If you don't want to give her cow's milk, try to breastfeed your daughter at least until her second birthday—or give her soy formula, not soy "milk" or drink, which is lower in fat and other essential ingredients. When she's two, offer her calcium-fortified soy drink. When it's time for solid food, give her mashed tofu, beans, and lentils, and finely chopped nuts and seeds. Call your local public health office for menu and recipe suggestions.*

Q: My kids gleefully drag home sacks of candy on Halloween. Should I let them gobble their goodies all at once and be done with it? If I dole out their candy, it seems to last forever!

A: *A one-night feed is easier on a child's teeth than eating the candy gradually over several days, but bingeing isn't a practice I encourage! Most kids get candy on a regular basis. Suggest they spread out their stash, perhaps eating something once a day, after dinner. Candy is easier on teeth when it's eaten at mealtime because there's likely to be a drink and plenty of saliva to rinse away the sugar. Dinnertime is also close to bedtime, when teeth should get a thorough brushing and flossing.*

Q: I know some kids with allergies to certain foods. I've heard peanut allergies can be serious—even lethal. Do you think schools should be peanut-free?

A: *Peanuts are one of the foods most likely to cause an extreme allergic reaction. Kids allergic to peanuts may experience a rapid swelling of the tongue and throat, and constriction of the airways in their lungs. While this "anaphylactic shock" is probably too rare to warrant peanut-free schools, it should be taken seriously. Some school boards have adopted guidelines to prevent and manage the problem. They suggest children at risk should eat only foods they bring from home, and avoid getting too close to other children who are eating the problem food. A child can have an allergic reaction after simply touching or smelling the food to which she's allergic! That means all children need to learn about allergies. Teachers of kids with life-threatening allergies must be trained to recognize a reaction and inject the medicine a child needs to stop the reaction. For more information, contact your local allergy or asthma information association and check that your child's school is up to date on this issue.*

Q: You put lots of emphasis on choosing vegetables and fruit. What about the pesticides commonly used on them? I worry about pesticide residues, yet I've heard organic produce isn't worth the extra cost.

A: *Health authorities monitor pesticide residues on fresh produce as much as possible, although studies show there's a wide variation in residues left on both domestic and imported foods. Wash firm fruits and vegetables in warm water and briefly soak leafy green vegetables in cold water. To be perfectly safe, peel produce, especially if you plan to make baby food. Certified organic fruit and vegetables are similar nutritionally to other produce, but they're usually free of pesticide residues. It's still important to wash them because natural fertilizers carry bacteria.*

Q: What do you think of the latest packaged lunch and snack kits that come with crackers, cheese, candy, and other goodies? My daughter begs for them.

A: *If you compare the price-per-weight with other foods, those cute packages are outrageously expensive. As packages within packages, they're not very kind to the environment, either. Why not buy one and help your daughter use it as a template for her own special lunches? You'll save money in the long run by buying your own food and packing it in reusable containers or small plastic bags. You'll be able to improve on quality, too. Go on a label-reading trip with your daughter and choose high-quality crackers, cheese, colorful veggies, and tasty meat—preferably nitrate-free. Show her that ingredients are always listed by weight, with the main ingredient at the top. Instead of candy bars, choose cookies with lots of grains and fruit. Have fun!*

GUIDELINES FOR BALANCED EATING

Daily Amounts Are Approximate – Follow Your
Appetite for a Variety of Healthy Foods!

GRAIN PRODUCTS

Sample serving: 1 slice of bread, 1 tortilla, ¾ cup (175 mL) dry cereal, ½ cup (125 mL) hot cereal, ½ cup (125 mL) pasta or rice, ½ muffin, bagel, hot dog bun, or hamburger bun

Pregnant or Breastfeeding: 5 to 12 servings

Babies 6* to 12 months: 4 to 8 tablespoons (60 to 125 mL) iron-fortified infant cereal

Toddlers 1 to 2½: 4 or more "child-size" servings (½ regular serving size)

Preschoolers 2½ to 6: 5 or more "child-size" servings

Children 6 to 12: 5 or more servings

Teenagers: 5 to 12 servings

VEGETABLES & FRUIT

Sample serving: 1 medium potato, tomato, carrot, pear, apple, banana, ½ cup (125 mL) broccoli, peas, squash, yam, grapes, ½ cup (125 mL) juice or tomato sauce, 1 cup (250 mL) leafy greens

Pregnant or Breastfeeding: 5 to 10 servings

Babies 6* to 12 months: 4 to 8 tablespoons (60 to 125 mL) mashed cooked vegetables and mashed or finely chopped fruit

Toddlers 1 to 2½: 4 or more "child-size" servings (½ regular serving size)

Preschoolers 2½ to 6:	5 or more "child-size" servings
Children 6 to 12:	5 or more servings
Teenagers:	5 to 10 servings

MILK & ALTERNATIVES

Sample serving:	1 cup (250 mL) milk, ⅔ cup (175 mL) plain yogurt, 1 finger-size piece of cheese 3 x 1 x 1 inch (7.5 x 2.5 x 2.5 cm), 2 slices of cheese, ¼ cup (60 mL) tofu made with calcium, or 1 cup (250 mL) calcium-fortified soy drink
Pregnant or Breastfeeding:	3 to 4 servings
Babies 6* to 12 months:	Breast milk or iron-fortified formula "on demand," about 3 to 4 cups (750 mL to 1 L)
Toddlers 1 to 2½:	3 or more "child-size" servings (½ regular serving size)
Preschoolers 2½ to 6:	2 full cups of milk, plus 1 "child-size" serving of another milk product or alternative
Children 6 to 12:	2 to 3 servings
Teenagers:	3 to 4 servings

MEAT & ALTERNATIVES

Sample serving:	1 "deck of cards" size piece of meat, fish, or poultry, 1 egg, ⅓ to ½ cup (75 to 125 mL) tofu, cooked dried beans or lentils, or 2 tablespoons (30 mL) peanut butter or hummus
Pregnant or Breastfeeding:	2 to 3 servings

Babies 6* to 12 months:	⅓ to ½ cup (75 to 125 mL) cooked minced meat, fish, poultry, dried beans, lentils, tofu (may include hummus, and the yolk *only* of 1 egg)
Toddlers 1 to 2½:	2 "child-size" servings (½ regular serving size)
Preschoolers 2½ to 6:	2 to 3 "child-size" servings
Children 6 to 12:	2 servings
Teenagers:	2 to 3 servings

*Babies may be ready for solid food as early as 4 months.

7

The Joy of Exercise

Nature beckons us to move to the rhythms of falling rain
and rushing streams, to the moon's tug on the tides.

You connect with your baby through movement, even before he's born. As he floats inside your womb, his every move assures you. After he's born, you instinctively rock and sway with him when he fusses. Motion comforts him. As the years go by, activity shapes your child—physically, mentally, emotionally.

You'll marvel at your baby's boundless energy. You'll be even more amazed at the way his body adapts to activity as he's growing up. He'll use his muscles and make them strong. His bones will become dense and sturdy as he walks, climbs, and runs. But nature is pragmatic: What we don't use, we lose. Bodies adapt to inactivity, too. If your child's days are filled with television, video games, computers, and car rides, he may not realize his full potential for strength and vitality.

With sedentary living, people of all ages often gain more fat than muscle. Today's adults burn 800 calories a day *less* than adults did 30 years ago—and our kids are right there beside us, jockeying for the remote. With each new generation, children are less active than their parents were during childhood. That coincides with kids getting taller and heavier on average, and more and more of them becoming overly fat. It's not a simple case of cause and effect. Inactive children may gain extra weight, but the reverse can also be true. Extra weight can make a child less active, especially if he feels self-conscious playing sports, has trouble keeping up with the others, or tends to be the last one picked for the team. When kids retreat to the sidelines, it's even easier for them to gain extra fat.

145

Sometimes, well-meaning adults tell a heavy child he needs more exercise than other kids do. That's not fair—and it's not true, either! *Everybody* benefits from physical activity—it shouldn't be optional for thin kids and mandatory "punishment" for heavier ones. Too many adults have come to see exercise as therapy. Kids deserve better. Shifting the focus from "exercise that's good for you" to the "fun of active living" allows children to see activity as a natural, pleasurable aspect of each day.

Feeling Good with Active Living

Pick up a pencil and squeeze it as hard as you can, all the time breathing normally. Now release the pencil. The muscles in your hand will feel soft, warm, and more relaxed than before you picked it up. When you exercise, your muscles contract and relax, releasing tension. After exercise, your entire body can feel warm and rested.

"Runner's high" isn't limited to runners. Any steady, moderately brisk aerobic activity can trigger the brain's release of "endorphins," making you feel somewhat euphoric. Exercise—especially in activities that require concentration—can also take your attention away from everyday worries. Some people repeat mantras or listen to music while they exercise to make their spirits soar!

Active living is a way of life, rather than something you have to do. It means taking every opportunity to move. Standing if you don't have to sit. Walking if you don't have to stand. Walking faster if there's no need to stroll. Active living can make you feel so good you'll want to move even more! It yields immediate benefits, helping you and your child feel vibrant, energetic, and confident—*now*.

It can also prevent future health problems, but kids tend not to look that far ahead.

Active living means enjoying recreation for its own sake rather than for a far-off health goal. Before I had kids of my own, I learned something as I watched a family hike in the mountains. As the parents trudged up the trail, their nine-year-old son amused himself by repeatedly forging ahead, and then retracing his steps. His mom and dad managed to keep an eye on him while letting the boy move at his own pace. My children also enjoyed the freedom to explore within safe limits. For me, walking outdoors is recreation at its best, allowing parents and kids to "re-create" themselves—body, mind, and soul.

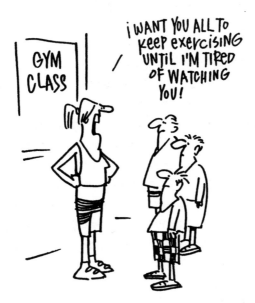

You don't have to be an athlete to bring up strong, active kids. I failed volleyball in the fourth grade because I couldn't hit the ball over the net, and I'm still not much of a swimmer! All it takes to raise active kids is a sense of fun, a simple pleasure in moving your body, and an appreciation of the outdoors.

This chapter is about building active living into *your* daily family life. Just as you offer your child healthy food and sit down to eat with him, you can set the stage for active living—and participate yourself. And just as it's not fair to tell a child certain foods will make him fat, it's not right to tell him exercise will make him slim! Like good food, active living promotes a healthy body weight, but it won't magically mold a child into any desired shape. Active living has the power to show your child what his body can do. It will also help prepare him for many of the challenges he'll face. What a confidence-builder! We can encourage *all* kids to be active—not because they need improvement, but because they deserve the best of what life has to offer.

Staying Safe while Keeping Active

While you're pregnant, let your credo be "moderation." Overdoing it can leave you feeling breathless. While this may not hurt you, it's important to maintain a steady flow of oxygen to your unborn baby. Women who exercise too strenuously can deliver low birth-weight babies who are at risk for several health problems. Experts also advise against exercising on your back after the fourth month of pregnancy. This helps avoid too much pressure on the large blood vessels—something that can interfere with your circulation.

Be sure to talk to your doctor before starting any new activity. Take it particularly easy during the first trimester if you weren't very active before pregnancy—overheating can interfere with critical stages of your baby's development. Even if you're very fit, ease off during the third trimester when your baby's growth needs are greatest.

Pregnancy brings new meaning to the term "safe sex"! After the fourth month, use positions that don't require you to lie flat on your back. Throughout your pregnancy, find new ways to enjoy intimacy without putting a strain on your body. You and your partner can cuddle and touch each other in ways that please you both, staying close even when you don't have intercourse. Ask your doctor how close to delivery it's safe to have intercourse, and how soon you can resume having sex after your baby's birth.

Stop any activity right away if you experience contractions or pain, or if there are changes in the way the baby moves. Let your doctor know what's happening.

The Infant – Your Personal Trainer

Early one morning while pushing Sarah in her stroller, I met a fellow who said, "I see you're out walking with your boss." Yes, babies tend to dictate our schedules! It's a good thing they're portable. Women all over the world carry infants on their chests or backs to satisfy their babies' needs for closeness, security, and action. A comfortable baby carrier, a sturdy stroller or carriage, and a safety-certified infant car seat can be your tickets to freedom.

Staying active is good for you *and* your baby. Physical activity can help you get your strength back after childbirth and cope with the stresses of being a new mom. It can also help regulate your appetite and body weight. If you're active, you'll sleep more soundly during those scarce hours when your baby's resting.

After pregnancy, take your time getting back in shape. If you exercise strenuously too soon after childbirth, you may find yourself "grounded" with stiff, sore muscles. When you exercise vigorously, a breakdown product from the fuel you burn can affect the flavor of your milk. While this substance won't harm your baby, you may want to minimize its effect. To do this, feed him right before you exercise, then wait at least an hour and a half after your workout before you feed him again.

Fueling Fitness

If your child ever darts into the street, you'll sprint after him at amazing speed. Your muscles store tiny amounts of a special fuel for emergencies like that. Your main sources of fuel are fat—stored all over the body—and sugar. Your blood contains sugar, with more of it readily available from "glycogen," a starchy material stored in the muscles and liver. While most activities require both fat and sugar in the fuel mix, steady brisk "aerobic" activity can help you burn more fat and less sugar by delivering oxygen to your working muscles.

If you exercise too strenuously to get enough oxygen to your muscles, your "aerobic" activity becomes "anaerobic"—literally "without oxygen." This means your body has to break down more glycogen to make sugar. As glycogen breaks down, a waste product called "lactic acid" collects in your muscles. Lactic-acid buildup can be painful—you may get a stitch in your side, or feel stiff and sore. Lactic acid can also make a mother's milk taste sour. You can minimize the buildup by exercising at a comfortable pace without becoming breathless.

Stretching before and after any type of exercise helps prevent lactic-acid buildup in the muscles. It can also help prevent injuries, particularly in activities such as squash and racquet ball that require fast movements with lots of stops and starts, and side-to-side motions.

Taking your baby for a daily walk can set a lifelong pattern for active living. You may think you're the one getting all the exercise, but your baby's connecting with Nature, too. Dressed for the weather, you can both enjoy being in touch with the sun, the wind, and the rain—a constantly changing world of new experiences. Right from the start, talk to your infant as you share your walk. He'll respond with coos and gurgles in no time!

Babies don't need special exercise programs, but they do need a chance to lie on their tummies as well as their backs. Today's infants are put on their backs to minimize the chance of suffocation as they sleep. That means they often don't spend enough time on their tummies for equal muscle development. As you cuddle and play with your baby, put him on his tummy, perhaps across your lap or on your chest as you recline. "Tummy time" helps babies with head and neck control, as well as arm and hand development. Make sure your little one has some "tummy time" each day—but never leave him on his tummy unattended.

A nursing baby can go almost anywhere. Help yours become accustomed to car travel early and he'll enjoy tagging along. Take a gentle hike. Go camping. As we prepared for Sarah's first weekend away at age three months, we groaned at the volume of clothing, diapers, and equipment that had become "basic necessities." But once the car was packed, it felt good to forget about housework for a while and recapture the delight of watching sunsets and taking long walks on the beach. I loved nursing Sarah outdoors, introducing my little girl to Nature's beauty.

The Older Baby – Moving Moments

In just a few months, a baby learns to roll over, sit up, stand, jump, crawl, walk, and sometimes climb! Never again will he experience so many "firsts" in such a short time. Your baby will work hard at progressing from one moving moment to the next.

All you have to do is make it safe and easy for him to do what comes naturally.

Let your baby follow his inclination to move in safe, spacious areas, continuing to put him on his tummy for a while each day until he learns to crawl. Dress him in comfortable clothing that won't restrict his movements. Older babies become Mr. Wiggles: It's nothing but fun to doff a glove here and a sock and shoe there! Babies who are old enough to sit can see, hear, and reach for new things as they enjoy the wider world. Branches in the park, fruit in the supermarket, other children, and entertaining dogs are all worth a lunge and a grab. So what's really happening here? All of this wriggling and jiggling, kicking and reaching, and grabbing and hoisting helps keep your curious baby's body and brain active.

Your baby may enjoy riding in a musical swinging baby seat, but fasten that safety belt. Let him star in his own baby bouncer ballet—but mount it securely. Your little one can dance on his toes while you stay on yours. No baby should be left unsupervised—staying nearby means you can talk to your child as he gurgles and laughs. There are plenty of toys and gadgets designed to help a baby explore his surroundings, but the greatest gift will be the time you spend playing with him.

Make your house "child-friendly" (I like that term better than "childproof") so your baby can crawl and pull himself around with no danger from breakables, sharp objects, household chemicals, or exposed electrical outlets. Even when you take precautions, an older baby needs constant supervision. Babies originated the phrase "going concern." One recall of child safety equipment found that probing fingers and repeated shaking could release the locking mechanism of some stairway gates, exposing the child to a potentially dangerous fall.

Infant walkers—those wheeled seats that let babies scoot around the house—were finally banned in many places after little riders suffered broken bones, burns, and even death. You may not see them in stores anymore, but they're still passed from one unsuspecting parent to another. Apart from being dangerous, an infant walker can delay your baby's motor development: Seeing his own feet improves a child's coordination. When he's ready, let your baby move on his own steam. He'll get a chance to use his muscles—and you'll have an easier time keeping him out of harm's way.

The Toddler – Poetry in Slow Motion

Your toddler can move like lightning around the house—especially if you're on the phone! But when he decides to climb out of his stroller and push it himself, you'll experience life in slow motion. When walks with your little one stop being invigorating, it's time to find other ways to be active—both together and apart. Doing something alone isn't selfish: It's hard to be a good parent if you're feeling grouchy and out of shape. Study after study shows that, in the long term, active parents have active kids.

Schedule outings to the park with your partner or friend. One person can supervise one or two toddlers at play while the other briskly walks or jogs around the perimeter. If you have an infant, take him along in a carriage or baby jogger. If you can arrange for an occasional sitter, taking a walk alone or with another adult can provide a "mental health" break. Imagine being alone with your thoughts for a while, or having an entire conversation with no interruptions!

Your toddler may also enjoy riding in a bicycle trailer on a quiet path, or in a backpack while you hike or cross-country ski. When you dress him for the outing, keep in mind that you'll be exercising, not him! Sadly, some tykes have suffered serious frostbite on faces, hands, and feet during otherwise-happy outings with Mom and Dad. A hat helps prevent heat loss when the weather's cool and sunstroke when it's hot. Always shade your child's eyes from the sun's glare—they're much more sensitive to ultraviolet light than adult eyes.

Some games are fun, indoors and out. Hide-and-seek offers plenty of bending, stretching, and running. Hide something special for your child to find and collect in a bucket: Socks and mittens work just fine, as long as there are enough items to hold your child's interest. Create a "popcorn" game by scrunching up pieces of white paper and spreading them on a towel. Folding it together, gently start to shake it, opening it slowly as you do. Let the "popcorn" fly—then pick it up and start over. Cardboard boxes make great toys, especially when they're large enough for you and your toddler to clamber in. Move your arms furiously as you "Row, row, row your boat, gently down the stream!" Think like a child and memories of active games will come flooding back.

Pools are wonderful places for parents and tots to splash and play. When my daughter Erica was a toddler, we went to a swim class where parents were shown how to put their little ones under water. The babies went along with it, but the toddlers spluttered and screamed. The morning after the first class, I opened my eyes to see Erica's little face right next to mine saying, "I'll blow bubbles, but don't put me undah da waddah!" I promised I wouldn't, right on the spot. We continued to enjoy visits to the pool—and Erica learned to swim when she was ready.

The American Academy of Pediatrics no longer recommends swimming lessons for children under the age of four, and experts now advise against dunking babies and toddlers under water. It doesn't make them "drownproof"—in fact, parents can get a false sense of security if they think their tiny tots can "swim" a few strokes. Drowning is a leading cause of injury and death for youngsters, and U.S. drowning rates are highest among toddlers aged one through two.

The Preschooler – Your Junior Athlete

One winter, my husband introduced the girls and me to downhill skiing. At 37, I was overly cautious. At two and a half, Erica had a short attention span. But at five, Sarah had reached the perfect teachable moment. Older preschoolers are built for sports. They're well coordinated and able to follow simple directions. They don't mind falling down, and they'll patiently try something again and again. They *love* to play and think that's what sports are all about (they should be!). On special occasions, the best gift you can give your preschooler is action gear such as balls of various sizes, a tricycle (and later, a bicycle), skates, or a swing set.

Your preschooler needs close supervision to keep him safe—but his confidence will soar when you let him do things his way. Don't discourage a child from being adventurous at playgrounds and water slides if you can let him "go for it" safely. Rather than saying, "That slide's too high for you!" climb up behind him, stationing someone at the bottom if there's any danger of a rough landing. At the ski hill, skip skiing with your child between your legs, and show him how to slide solo down short, gentle slopes with his hands on his knees. He'll soon learn how to stop by himself, gaining a wonderful sense of control. Go outside and toss a beach ball with your preschooler, or chase a soccer ball around the yard (knowing "the rules" isn't important). Physical games are lots of fun, but no tickling, please! Respect your child's body as you respect your own—tickling can be torture. Teach your child the active games you played as a child. There are dozens that need no special equipment. Remember tag and hopscotch?

Keep a preschooler from getting bored on a long walk or hike: Help him collect leaves or acorns, count flowers, or look for "fairy houses" along the way. Collecting stones is permissible on many beaches—although I don't recommend it on steep trails. One day we wondered why our young nephew kept lagging behind, only to find he was filling his backpack with rocks the size of a fist!

The Primary School Child – A Team Player

Yesterday, he was a little kid; today, he's a schoolboy! Yesterday, you taught him about sharing and cooperative play; now he'll learn about competition, too. He'll take gym classes and run races. He may be assigned to a house team where he'll play sports with kids from other grades. Perhaps he'll join a soccer league and come home wearing a uniform. After one practice, he'll tell you his team's the best!

Physical education may be your child's most important subject in elementary school. Regular activity helps kids relax while keeping them alert. It improves their ability to concentrate and solve problems. Vigorous physical activity actually stimulates brain cell production. It also allows kids to blow off steam so they're less likely to be restless in the classroom or aggressive on the playground. Studies show that attending good gym classes on a daily basis can boost self-esteem and help kids get good grades.

Of course, physical education programs vary in quality—and in some schools, they don't exist! Give your child's teacher and principal your wholehearted support for at least 30 minutes of daily physical education. Ask about the balance between cooperation and competition, and about the way classes are structured to keep kids having fun and on the move. If your child looks forward to his gym class, his school probably has a good program.

As you send your child to school for the first time, you may wonder how he'll handle competition. Do kids need to experience "the school of hard knocks," or should we try to protect them from losing? With primary school children, the question at the end of every game should be, "Did everyone have fun?" rather than "Which team won?" As kids get older, however, the thrill of winning a game or contest can be empowering, and it's frustrating if parents discourage friendly competition. Canadian fitness expert and author Gordon Stewart likes to see a child *strive* to win without getting attached to winning. A child who does this—who really concentrates and tries hard—can accept losing a game if his parents and coach remain upbeat and encouraging. There's no better way to teach sportsmanship—surely one of the most practical things a child can learn.

While organized sports can be fun for kids, younger children need plenty of unstructured play. After a snack and a chat, my girls often dashed off to meet a friend, although they sometimes just walked into their rooms and closed their doors. Imaginative play—whether it's boisterous or sedate—offers more release from tension than sitting in front of the tube. If you find your child spends too much time watching TV or playing on the computer, ask him to turn it off. You don't have to tell him how to amuse himself—finding something else to do is his job! If your child goes to after-school daycare, discuss activity options with your care provider.

You'll also do your child a favor if you let him walk or ride his bike whenever it's safe and practical, rather than driving him everywhere. If *you* sometimes walk or pedal instead of driving, he'll be less likely to say, "No fair!" when you suggest it to him.

The Preteen – At a Turning Point

Active kids have higher self-esteem than sedentary kids and are less likely to start smoking—a habit that often begins in the preteen years. Unfortunately, kids often start to get less active around the fourth grade—and get progressively less active as they get older. It takes the cooperation of parents, teachers, coaches, and maybe even celebrities to reverse this unhealthy trend. In the meantime, encourage *your* preteen to stay active.

Gym classes are important. They not only affect what kids do at school, but also influence what they do *after* school. Kids are more likely to lead active lives if they have a good attitude about gym class and feel competent participating. Teachers and parents can help a child of any ability develop a positive outlook. Check to see if building self-esteem is a priority in your child's gym classes. Watch for signs that everyone in the class has fun—not just the star athletes.

Kids who enjoy vigorous activities tend to spend less time in passive pursuits. Still, most kids show a very human tendency to "take it easy." Recognizing this, you may want to set limits on watching TV and playing video games. Some experts worry about video games even more than television. Because they hook kids by involving them in the action, video games are fast, exciting, and competitive, appealing to kids who might otherwise go outside and round up their neighborhood buddies for some spirited play.

Preteen girls seem to need more encouragement to be active than boys of the same age, but the extra support is worth the effort. Participation in sports can have unexpected payoffs for girls. Physically active girls are half as likely to engage in early sexual activity as their physically inactive peers. Studies also suggest physically active girls are more likely to use contraception than girls with less body awareness.

How can you encourage preteens to be active? Help them plan outings and birthday parties at the park, bowling alley, skating rink, water slides, or community pool. Active parties are always more fun than another round of movies. Family activities are also fun, but don't be surprised to hear a preteen say: "Do we *have* to go hiking today?" Many a kid this age groans at the words "family outing." Let your child occasionally invite a friend on a family excursion. On some days, let him make his own plans—or no plans at all. One couple I know revived their son's interest in family outings when they brought a new puppy into the family. Decorate your house with pictures of your child and his friends playing games and sports. Photos are terrific reminders of good times. They also help a child see himself as an active person.

Just when things are going relatively smoothly, you may come to a new hurdle. You've worked hard to teach your child that healthy kids come in all shapes and sizes, but now he has a teacher or coach who doesn't realize a young person can be fit and strong without appearing slim. The "fit or fat" myth can be especially hard on girls who enjoy gymnastics, dance, figure skating, or synchronized swimming—activities that place a high value on a slim appearance or a light body weight.

Olympic-level gymnasts are getting even smaller. They're now 6 inches (15 cm) shorter and nearly 20 pounds (9 kg) lighter than they were in the late '70s. Even the equipment has changed to favor smaller bodies! The problem isn't limited to elite athletes—ordinary kids also try to fit these tiny molds.

Imagine how it feels to be a preteen advised to lose several pounds for her sport, or to be a girl who loves to dance, only to be told she's too big for ballet! Some coaches give advice that fosters unhealthy living and low self-esteem. They don't mean to do it, but it happens. Get to know your child's coach, and don't be too shy to speak up.

The Young Teen – Struggling to Stay Real

In a recent study of 26,000 teens, more than half the girls were trying to lose weight, while a quarter of the boys wanted to gain it. During the term of the study, nearly half the kids of both sexes reported feeling irritable or depressed—emotional states that may have been linked to their attempts to change their bodies.

The early teen years are a time when kids often go to extremes. Some retreat to a world of daydreams. The more inactive they become, the less "at home" they feel in their bodies, perpetuating the cycle of inactivity. Some physical education teachers think they can motivate kids by weighing them, or using calipers or other instruments to estimate levels of body fat. Bad idea! To do so can make kids feel self-conscious, hurt, and angry. Even if the teacher's intentions are good—and they usually are—some kids will decide they hate gym and that being active is "stupid."

Meanwhile—whether the trigger is the fat test or the cultural milieu—some kids become obsessed with running to get thin or pumping iron to bulk up. For girls, overexercising can lead to a combination of three interrelated conditions: eating disorders such as anorexia, interrupted menstrual periods, and bone loss. When a girl's body fat levels drop too low—from overexercising and/or undereating—her periods stop. Estrogen levels drop, which in turn causes bones to lose calcium. This often happens to athletes and dancers, but it's also becoming increasingly common among average kids playing sports at school. Let your daughter know that if anything interrupts her periods, it's important to see a doctor. Don't delay. Even a few missed periods can make a difference to her bone mass. (Anorexic boys who overexercise can also compromise bone health.)

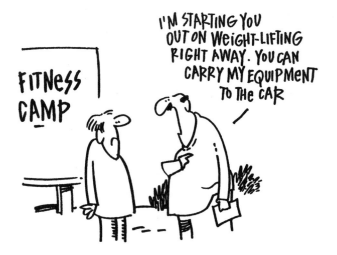

Boys who preoccupy themselves with bulking up their muscles can harm their health, too. Aside from a temptation to experiment with muscle-enhancing supplements, an overcommitment to weight training may leave no time or energy for other pastimes—not even healthy aerobic activities. Boys and girls who exercise obsessively are often afraid to stop. They would rather risk illness and injury than listen to their bodies' signals to slow down.

You can help your child by following a moderate, balanced lifestyle yourself. Invite your couch potato teen to join you for walks—it's a great way to share some time in a busy day. Ask your teenaged fitness fanatic to take a break with you at the beach or the park. Parents often underestimate the influence they have on their young teens. Teen health studies confirm that kids want strong connections with their parents. Teens who are close to one or both parents tend to be healthier than kids who lack this closeness. They also tend to be less likely to smoke, drink, or use drugs. Of course, that doesn't mean kids who are close to their parents never have problems. It just means that spending time with your child is always worthwhile.

The Older Teenager – Marching to His Own Drummer

Your older teen "has a life." In it, activity may play a lead role, a supporting part, or no part at all! If he's very active—blasting down trails on a mountain bike or taking jumps on his skateboard—safety may be your primary concern. On the other hand, if your older teenager spends all his time surfing the Net or hefting school books (it can happen!), you may be more worried about future coronaries than present concussions. (Parents always find *something* to worry about!)

Once your child has graduated from high school, he may never again play basketball or soccer. The kid who grew up with daily physical education may never set foot in a gym as a young adult. A recent study shows that by the time he's in his 30s, he may be as out of shape as age-mates who were less active as kids. Consider helping your child participate in lifestyle activities such as racquet sports, cycling, and skiing. It's great for kids to manage their own money from part-time jobs and allowances, but if you can afford to match their contributions for bikes, hiking boots, snowboards, and fitness-center fees, they may be less likely to miss out on worthwhile activities. Show your child how to develop a fitness plan and how to adapt it as his circumstances change in college or the workplace. Fitness and activity aren't a "program" to be followed, but a "lifestyle" with lifelong benefits.

What if your older teen shows no interest in exercise? I'd treat him as I would an adult with the same inclinations. Telling him to get off his duff won't motivate a teenager anymore than it will a coworker or friend! Invite him to be active in ways that spark his interest, perhaps taking a weekend away to explore a nearby town on foot or to visit a national park. If he enjoys himself, he may be willing to follow up with walks near home. As your child gets older, he'll notice the practical advantages of active living—such as gaining the stamina to take a trip, packing lots of action into each day.

If your child *is* active in sports, ensure that he has access to appropriate safety equipment. Young athletes are vulnerable to serious injuries. No one should ride a bike or play such sports as football or hockey without a helmet. I've heard kids use the excuse that protective padding for sports such as skateboarding or in-line skating is too expensive. You may wish to subsidize the cost. Of course, your child may decline protective gear for fear of appearing "uncool." The biggest safety obstacle for teenagers is their sense of invincibility.

Good running shoes protect kids from injury, too. Shin splints and sore heels aren't as dramatic as concussions or broken wrists, but they can keep kids out of commission just as long. Help your child budget for new runners once or twice a year. The soles often outlast the uppers, so help your teen notice when the uppers lose stability and strength.

The time may come when you look at your "grown-up" teenager and feel the same sense of wonder you did when you counted his tiny fingers and toes. Since the first time you held him in your arms, you've carried him in your heart—and you always will. Even before birth, he moved independently. Now, your teenager is getting ready to separate from you. Quite rightly, he has his *own* way of doing things. When you're 17, you don't think your parents know anything. When you're 21, you wonder how they learned so much in a few short years! Relax. If your child has enjoyed active living over the years, the seeds you've planted will probably grow strong roots.

Because You Asked about Active Living

Q: My friend's three-year-old son is much more muscular than our preschooler. What can my husband and I do to help Jason become fitter?

A: *If you suspect a problem in Jason's muscular development, be sure to take him to a pediatrician. At his age, fitness isn't a factor in muscle definition. A child who's particularly muscular at the age of three will have inherited that trait. If your doctor assures you Jason is developing normally, encourage your son in active play—swinging and climbing at the playground, playing tag and hide-and-seek. Keep the focus on fun rather than fitness. Heredity will influence Jason's build throughout life, but as he grows up, physical activity will also affect the way his muscles develop.*

Q: Active living sounds great, but will it help my chubby six-year-old become slimmer as she grows up? When is a child too heavy? I wonder if I should enroll my daughter in a program for overweight kids?

A: *Active living can help protect your little girl from putting on excess weight, but it won't necessarily make her slim. Encourage her to participate in activities she enjoys on a daily basis. A class in tumbling, skating, or dance may complement her active play nicely, as long as she enjoys it. Talk to your doctor privately about your concerns, so you can speak freely without hurting your daughter's feelings. Figuring out if a child is "too heavy" isn't easy. If your daughter is gaining weight faster than she's growing in height, your doctor may recommend a special program or refer you to a dietitian. I favor family-oriented programs that don't single out a child as the one with a "problem."*

Q: Like me, my teenaged daughter is "well-endowed"—and totally disinterested in sports. I think she'd benefit from an exercise program, but I know she's self-conscious about participating in activities that call attention to her figure.

A: *Talk to your daughter about activities she may enjoy—not to change her body, but to have fun and feel good. Perhaps you could do something together such as go to the gym or play badminton at the community center. The right undergarments and exercise clothing can help your daughter enjoy moving without feeling too self-conscious. Consider shopping together for sports bras. You both may be comfortable wearing two, one layered on top of the other. To encourage each other, consider logging your outings on the calendar or in a shared journal, noting such things as weather conditions and how you both feel after your activity. You may want to make a bargain to splurge on treats such as new sports socks or a bandana at the end of each month you've been active.*

Q: Paul, our 10-year-old, is small for his age. He's often the last one picked for school sports teams, but he doesn't want me to talk to the gym teacher.

A: *I suspect Paul isn't the only one who's uncomfortable with the way teams are picked. The same thing may be happening in other classes, too. Talk to someone you trust—a teacher, a principal, or someone active in the parents' association—and ask that the issue be brought up at a staff meeting with no names mentioned. I'm sure the teachers will have no trouble coming up with a fair way to pick teams, not only in gym class, but for other activities, too.*

Q: My daughter's about to leave home for college. She anticipates lots of starchy, high-fat foods in residence—and not enough time to run. She's heard about the "freshman 15"—pounds, that is! What can I tell her?

A: *Congratulate your daughter on anticipating something that catches a lot of students unaware. The workload tends to be heavier at college than in high school. If she puts off exercising until she "finishes" studying, she'll never get out the door! Help her plan to build activities into her schedule to boost her fitness and help her relax. Suggest that, as part of her orientation to college, she check out safe places to walk or run, and/or find a gym where she'll feel comfortable working out. She may need special exercise clothing or backup plans for changes in climate over the school term. She may also need some advice for choosing balanced meals and snacks at the cafeteria. Without a plan, it's very easy to overeat in cafeterias, where there are many things to choose from.*

8
The Essence of Ease

Nature replenishes us. Daily,
she bids us to rest and relax, repairing
the body and renewing the spirit.

In a treasured baby picture, my mother holds me against her cheek
to comfort me. Imagine my joy when Sarah wrote a poem in the
first grade that said: "My mother hugs me tight and I'm all right."
As your child grows up, don't you wish you could always be
there to make everything all right? While that's not possible, you
can help your child learn how to be at ease, and how to get the
encouragement and support she needs. That's what this chapter
is all about.

What does it mean to be "at ease"? For me, the phrase suggests
relaxation, comfort, freedom from pressure, and a certain "lightness"

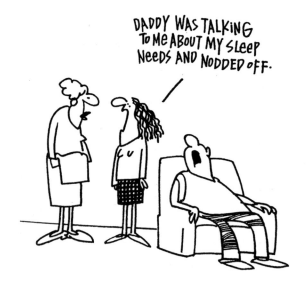

DADDY WAS TALKING
TO ME ABOUT MY SLEEP
NEEDS AND NODDED OFF.

of being. Life is so much better—and healthier—when we know how to relax and be easy.

Your ability to manage stress can even affect your weight. Without ease, it's difficult for you and your child to eat well and stay active. Yet if you don't eat well and stay active, your stress levels will climb even higher! When life is chaotic and rushed, it's unrealistic to expect eating to be moderate and relaxed. When we eat quickly, we don't pay much attention to the quantity or quality of our food. The problem compounds itself when we're too busy or too tired to exercise. As if that weren't enough, stress can cause a body to hoard fat. During and immediately after stressful situations, some people produce more fat-building enzymes, making it easier for the body to store fat, particularly around the waist.

Stress and time pressures can also be hard on your self-esteem. When there's not enough time to do everything well, you may begin to feel you can't do *anything* well. It's hard to shift priorities when you can't find time to stop and think. I remember the gentler pace of the '60s. My professors predicted that new advances in technology would bring more leisure time. I expected to own a helpful robot by now—not a slave-driving computer! The weird thing about technology is that it makes us feel important while simultaneously burdening us with more responsibilities. We brag about the number of e-mails and voice-mails that flood in. We rush to scoop up faxes, accepting other people's priorities as our own. In the middle of meetings and traffic jams, beepers and cell phones demand attention. I recently watched a woman talk on the phone as she strolled through a toy store, oblivious to her child's appeals to, "Look, Mom! Mo-om, *look!*"

Robot fantasies aside, the future is now—and leisure time is disappearing rather than increasing. Pollsters conclude the average couple spends only 20 minutes a day together. Studies suggest busy couples typically put their children's needs ahead of their own. Despite that, more than half of the parents surveyed feel that, by the end of a typical day, they haven't spent enough time with their kids. They're probably right. According to one study, today's parents spend 40 percent less time with their children than parents did in the '50s. A recent newspaper article about working parents showed a photo of a mother staring intently at her computer screen while her preschool daughters looked on. The message? Mom doesn't have to spend more than 10 hours a day at the office, because she can work at her home computer after dinner!

Children of workaholics often have highly programmed lives. Tots dash from violin lessons to ballet to language tutoring to piano practice to martial arts to gymnastics. Like any repetitive behavior, hurrying and cramming become habits. You can find yourself rushing your children just to go to preschool, exercise class, or a friend's house, all the time chirping, "Quick, kids. We're late!" If you start your day by jamming a child's arms into her coat and flinging stuff into the car, it's time to step back and reevaluate.

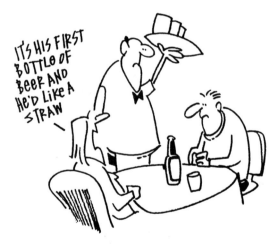

This chapter will help your family become more stress-resistant. Start with your own life and, like the ripples in a pond, the good vibes will spread to other family members. Life will always be unpredictable and complicated, but it will help if you can catch yourself when you're rushing needlessly or starting to feel tense. Take a deep breath, slow down, relax. You *can* learn to respond to stressful situations before you become irritable or tired. And you can teach your kids to do the same.

Responding to Stress in Pregnancy

Do you ever paste a smile on your face and say everything's fine, while underneath that placid demeanor, tiny muscles are clenching, adrenaline is surging, and your brain is shrieking: "I can't take it anymore!" It's easy to fool others, but you can't fool your own body. If you're pregnant, your unborn baby will share the biochemical soup of your anxiety. There's evidence that pregnant women who often feel stressed-out may program their unborn babies' nervous systems to overreact to stress. If ever there was a time to ease more relaxation into your life, this is it!

Stress isn't something that happens outside your body. It results when you react—rather than respond—to life's everyday trials. Can you handle daily pressures without relying on medications, alcohol, or food to release the tension? Do you notice when you feel pressured *before* that headache or backache develops? Do you make a conscious effort to release muscle tension often during the day by stretching or moving around? It helps if you're able to let people around you know how you feel and what you need. It's not easy to live a healthy life without support from family and friends.

If you relax by smoking or drinking, this is the time to consider safer ways to cope. Your doctor or prenatal

instructor can help you find the support you need. Don't
be embarrassed—be proud of yourself for asking!

The Infant – Dream Weaver

Ah, sleep! You need it. Your baby needs it. Getting enough of it is
a prime goal for new parents. When you're tired, nothing's "easy."

Babies' sleep patterns vary tremendously. Some newborns sleep
or drowse for 16 hours a day in two- to four-hour stints. Others
sleep only 10 hours out of 24. I found my first baby didn't sleep
much during the day unless she was pushed in a carriage or
driven in the car. As an inexperienced mom, I didn't realize a
baby isn't always fully awake when she makes a noise. Babies can
cry out and make all sorts of sounds during light sleep. Maybe
I was sometimes too quick to pick her up—but maybe not. As
she grew up, Sarah never seemed to need a lot of sleep, and she
still doesn't.

New parents dream of the time when their babies will sleep
through the night. Your baby may start to sleep longer at three
months, or she may still wake up at night when she's a toddler.
Some babies sleep through at four months only to experience
interrupted nights again at nine months when they're well into
teething, or getting ready to crawl or walk.

Canadian child development specialist Judith Banfield says
there are no "black or white" answers when it comes to sleep patterns. It's less stressful for parents to accept their baby's unique
"sleep nature" and find ways to adjust to it, rather than try to
correct it. If your baby gets you up frequently during the night,
Banfield suggests turning your bedside clock to the wall so you
don't find yourself timing your baby's "wake-up" calls!

There's no harm in trying to maintain a quiet household during the night. When your infant wakes for nighttime changing and feeding, caring for her quickly and quietly sends the message that nights are for sleeping. Don't turn on any bright lights, talk, or play the way you would during the day. With luck, your gentle touch will be all the assurance she'll need to fall asleep again!

You can expect your dream baby to disturb *your* sleep. Unfortunately, sleep deprivation tends to disrupt every aspect of your life. Your body needs sleep to repair, restore, and rejuvenate itself. Without enough sleep, your immune system weakens, exposing you to colds and flu. You become less alert, which can affect your driving. You get irritable, which can affect your relationships. Fatigue can mess with your appetite, too, making it hard to control your weight. You may find yourself focusing on "down" moments rather than "ups."

Make rest a priority and the entire household will benefit. Take a nap when your newborn drops off to sleep during the day. Show housework tender loving neglect! The cobwebs can wait—you'll have more energy once you're fully recovered from childbirth and your baby has a more regular routine. A daily walk will help you sleep well, but strenuous exercise close to bedtime can keep you wired for two hours or more.

All new moms need a support system. A diaper service for a month or two makes a great baby gift (drop a hint to someone close). Calling in a babysitter or housekeeper for a few hours can help you recoup your energy after a sleepless night.

You'll find that when you're tense, your baby will also be tense. There's no getting around it—you're a team now. When Erica was eight weeks old, we moved to a new town. Nursing was impossible the morning the moving van came. My neighbor invited us over—tearful mom and howling babe—and tried to make us comfortable in a rocking chair in her quiet bedroom. Erica still screamed. It's not easy to relax during stressful times. Now I "practice" relaxing regularly, so I can find serenity when I need it!

The Older Baby – Easy Rider

I once overheard a new mother saying, "Life is hell at our house at dinnertime!" As a new mom, I found the comment reassuring. I hadn't even admitted to myself that it was tough cooking meals during the baby's fussy time. Once, I tried to throw a dinner party and my guests arrived to find me pacing up and down the street behind Sarah's carriage. Knowing the situation was normal helped me laugh it off. Parents need to spend time with other new parents who are sharing the same experiences at the same time.

I love speaking to groups of young parents about infant nutrition—even though I can never count on my audience's full attention! With one ear cocked in my direction, the parents are tuned to their babies, occasionally nursing, rocking and shushing, reaching out to fix a toy for a passing toddler. New-parent groups offer good opportunities to develop child-rearing skills. As well as learning from visiting experts, parents learn from each other, developing lasting social networks. The babies in the audience get what they need most: close contact with their moms and dads in a relaxing, supportive situation.

Older babies grow and develop quickly, learning new skills at an amazing rate. The best way to keep them happy and at ease is to maintain a predictable yet flexible routine for meals, snacks, playtime, and bedtime. While you may have taken your infant everywhere you went, consider occasionally leaving an older baby with a trusted sitter. Older babies often prefer their own beds and bedtime routines to being tucked in somewhere new. A familiar blanket and stuffed toy can help an older baby feel at home when you travel.

It's never too soon to start building your child's confidence. Your baby will feel secure when she can count on you to understand her needs—to know when she's hungry and when she's had enough food; to know when she needs to be changed, cuddled, or rocked to sleep.

Child-rearing experts still debate how parents should respond to a child's crying in the night. Some recommend letting her cry herself to sleep, while others suggest bringing her into your bed. There's a wide range of options in between. Your baby may be reassured if you cover her up and pat her for a while, speaking or singing softly. Or she may cry even harder because she needs to be in someone's arms! Some parents pace the floor or rock the baby until she settles down. Helping your little one feel loved and secure as she drops off to sleep is not always easy. If you find yourself at the end of your rope and feel you're likely to be impatient with your baby, she may be better off crying for a while. Partners can sometimes spell each other off when one loses patience, and a visiting grandparent can really come in handy. The overall goal for the family should be to preserve the parents' sanity while maintaining loving feelings toward the baby.

The Toddler – It's My Potty and I'll Cry if I Want To!

I clearly remember my first child's toilet training. In the end (pardon the pun), I wrote her a story in which her bottom was an animated character. I don't remember anything about my second child's toilet training. Not a single detail. With the right attitude and perspective, you can see each stage a child goes through as a normal learning experience.

Take the "terrible two's"—*please!* Two-year-olds spend their days saying "*No!*" with the occasional (or not so occasional) tantrum tossed in. Children of that age are more fun if you look upon their behavior as an important developmental step, rather than a dreadful stage. Your two-year-old is beginning to see herself as a separate, independent being. That's a good thing—even if mealtimes require superhuman patience!

Progressing toward Relaxation

Choose a quiet, private place to lie on a mat, carpet, or firm mattress. Close your eyes, breathing deeply and naturally, inhaling energy through your nose, exhaling tension through your mouth. After three deep breaths, focus your attention on your right foot. Curl your toes for three seconds—hold, hold, hold ... *release*. Your foot will feel heavy and warm. Let it sink deeply into the floor or mattress. Repeat with your left foot. Continue to breathe deeply and naturally—in through the nose, out through the mouth—and let the tension leave your body. Focus on your right hand. Make a tight fist—one second, two seconds, three seconds ... *release*. Your hand will feel heavy and warm, as though it were sinking. Repeat with your left hand. Move your attention to your buttocks and then your shoulders, continuing your progressive clench and release of muscles. Finally, scrunch up the muscles in your face, and then let your face relax. After progressive relaxation, you can expect to feel like a soft, heavy rag doll.

Important note: Clench your muscles just enough to feel some tension, continuing to breathe normally as you do so. Hold the tension for a few seconds. Don't clench your toes if the muscles in your feet cramp easily. Instead, put your attention on each foot by gently moving it.

Maintain your sense of humor by making a point of relaxing often. "Progressive relaxation" is an easy way to reduce tension. Let your toddler join in by turning it into a game of "do this, do this, do that," letting her copy your moves. She'll giggle at the face-scrunching!

Your toddler's most wonderful quality is her ability to live in the moment. She'll play peek-a-boo until you're peeked right out. She'll never tire of a game or story. Make her laugh, and she'll think you're the wittiest person on earth. Your toddler will reacquaint you with the true meaning of play. Sometimes adults blur the line between play and work. Pure play is its own reward. A recent study of self-employed people concluded a huge percentage were so engrossed in their businesses, they had little time for anything else. Then there's the weekend athlete, so busy "working" on his golf swing or tennis serve, he forgets to have fun. Your toddler won't have any of those hang-ups. Play is central to children's development, giving them the chance to master new tasks and skills.

Establish a bedtime routine to help your toddler relax and get ready to sleep. Plan to spend at least 15 to 30 minutes, starting with a bath and ending with a story or soft music. This is a time for subtle lighting and a minimum of background noise. Let your toddler make some choices so she'll have a sense of control over the bedtime ritual. Perhaps she could choose between two pairs of pajamas, and pick one or two stuffed toys to take to bed. Let her select a reasonable number of stories. Aim for a nice quiet time together that doesn't feel rushed. Some children will need more time than others—they may fear being left alone in their rooms, or they may not fall asleep easily. Try to strike a balance between your child's needs and your own. Before *you* drift off to sleep, allow some "adult time" for you and your partner.

Practicing Quieting for Peace of Mind

Sit in a comfortable chair. Keep your back straight, feet flat on the floor, knees apart, hands resting on your thighs. Or sit cross-legged, with a pillow under your bottom to help keep your back straight. Close your eyes. Begin by noticing your breath without changing it. Now start to breathe slowly and deeply, down into your abdomen. If you've been tensing your abdominal muscles, release them. As you *inhale*, think the words "I am." As you *exhale*, think the word "relaxed." Continue to breathe slowly and deeply as you repeat in your mind, "I am ... relaxed." Do this exercise for three or four minutes—and repeat it as often as you can during your busy day. Gradually increase your "quieting" time or "meditation."

When your mind wanders, *let go* of each thought and refocus your attention on your breath. Don't dwell on distractions or impatiently push them away. Quieting isn't a problem to solve or a goal to reach. It's a break from the usual buzz in your life. Quieting won't put you in a trance, and it shouldn't put you to sleep. It allows you to be alert and relaxed at the same time.

When you're a parent, "quieting" can help keep your priorities straight. Having a special "quieting place"—complete with a pretty plant and a few favorite photos—will remind you to practice often. When your child's a toddler or preschooler, take her to your "quieting place" when she's upset. You may want to seat her on a small "calming" chair or cushion, next to yours—a peaceful place to regain her composure. Whenever a child yells or cries loudly, whisper to her or speak in a very low voice—she'll have to quiet down to hear you.

The Preschooler - Never Caught Napping

Most of the growth and development of your child's brain takes place *after* birth. During her first few years, much of the brain's circuitry will be formed by interactions between heredity and everyday experiences. Something like 50,000 genes are involved in the development of the nervous system. But "good genes" aren't enough to program the enormous number of brain circuits your child has the potential to develop. She also needs plenty of sights, sounds, smells, and tastes to stimulate her brain.

Positive early childhood experiences will help your child be the best she can possibly be. Happy moments stimulate the release of endorphins, the "feel good" brain chemicals that encourage the growth of nerve cells and the connections between them. Hormones released by high levels of stress can have the opposite effect, permanently impairing a child's intellectual and emotional growth. Kids from chaotic, unstable homes sometimes become so accustomed to a constant flow of adrenaline that they feel empty and bored when life *isn't* so hectic!

A variety of activities and experiences can be enriching, as long as a child's life isn't overly organized. It's good for pre-schoolers to play with friends and feel like part of a group. But there's nothing your preschooler would rather do than to spend time with *you*. "Quality" time has become a euphemism for spending 30 minutes with a child at the end of an exhausting day. Quantity counts, too. If you don't have enough time to relax with your child, it's not "quality" time, regardless of what you do together.

Let your child choose the activity and take the time to play. Create an imaginary village with building blocks. Haul out simple board games you enjoyed as a child. Walk to the library and choose a stack of books. Build a bedroom "fort" together—illuminated by flashlights—and read bedtime stories. Preschoolers still need their moms or dads to tuck them into bed, maintaining the closeness that began in infancy.

I know a woman who still regrets not having taken more time to play with her kids. Her line of work? She was a housewife. Her large home and garden took much of her time, and she raised, cooked, and preserved all her family's food. Whether you're a stay-at-home parent or a brain surgeon, your kids need you. And you need them! Find a way to drop some of your duties—and discover how good it feels to kick back with your family.

A child wants nothing more—or less—than her parents' full attention during part of every day. There'll always be other demands on your time, but when you're with your child, it's wonderful to be fully present. That's the true meaning of quality time.

The Primary School Child – Complete with Rechargeable Batteries

Realizing that my frame of mind affected the whole household, I started meditating when the kids were young. I remember finding a quiet corner of the house to sit and practice, trying to ignore the sound of little girls shouting to each other, "Where's Mom?" "She's upstairs! She doesn't want to be disturbed!" "What's she doing?" "She's meditating!" "When'll she be finished?" "*I don't know!*"

The girls weren't interested in "quieting," but they found it relaxing to look at books and color pictures. They also needed enough sleep to wake refreshed in the morning, so we tried to keep regular bedtimes. Even after they outgrew bedtime stories, I continued to tuck them in at night (sometimes we'd talk about things that never came up "in the light of day"). It's nice if the last words your child hears before falling asleep come from a loving parent rather than a TV program. Television viewing can be linked to sleep disturbances among primary school children, especially when the TV is in the child's bedroom. Disrupted sleep is more common when children watch a great deal of television, or view upsetting programs just before they fall asleep.

It's important for young children to know how to relax, but stress management involves more than that. Kids also need guidance in interacting with others. Children who are particularly compliant may get too much praise for being cooperative. With reinforcement like that, a child may never learn to be assertive. Make a point of teaching your child to speak up for herself, especially if you suspect she's inherited the "good behavior" gene!

Youngsters are often exposed to teasing and put-downs that can be devastating to their self-image. Encourage your child to talk about her day. If someone treated her unfairly ask, "How did that make you *feel?*" Then help her decide how to make her feelings and wishes known. Let her practice what she wants to say while you take the role of the other child or the teacher. That way, your child handles the situation, knowing you're behind her. Without giving your child the impression the world revolves around her, show her that she's important by teaching her how to give herself positive "self-talk." Even young children can learn to say: "I'm a good person who deserves to be heard!"

It may be difficult for you to give advice like that if your own self-esteem is shaky. If you catch yourself making self-disparaging remarks, stop and turn the criticism into a compliment. Rather than "I hate my hips!" try: "I have a womanly figure." Rather than "I screwed up again!" try: "I'm working too hard—I need a break." Once you master positive self-talk in *your* life, you can teach it to your child. If you hear her say, "I'm fat!" ask her why she's feeling down on herself and help her rephrase the remark. When kids say things like that, they usually mean, "I feel lousy today." None of us is perfect, but all of us have good qualities. Together with your child, start the day with some positive self-talk—and see how infectious good thoughts can be! Some schools are now teaching parents stress-reduction techniques they can share with their children. This initiative recognizes that people of all ages can benefit from positive self-talk, relaxed breathing, and pleasant visualizations.

The Preteen – Born Free!

At times, your older child may feel carefree. On other days, she'll seem to carry the weight of the world on her shoulders. Adults are often surprised to learn that children are concerned about big issues such as wars, environmental problems, and crime. Kids sometimes worry about their parents as much as their parents worry about them! They may fret about their moms and dads getting angry or sick, or splitting up.

You can buffer your child from some of the harsher realities of her world. Sometimes she'll need an advocate to go with her to discuss a problem at school or at a neighbor's (this is true of younger children, too). She'll never stop needing *you* to love her unconditionally—and she may appreciate a pet, often the most loyal supporter of all! Preteens still liked to be tucked into bed. One mom used to whisper in her sleeping son's ear: "You're the best! You're wonderful! You're a success!" He grew up to be a happy, healthy, self-confident man. Kids live up—or down—to the messages they hear.

The preteen years are an important time to foster mutual respect. Let your child know you *also* have needs—for rest, relaxation, encouragement, and support. It's empowering for a child to take on responsibilities around the house, to show kindness to others, and to bask in the glow of sincere appreciation. Remind your child about others' birthdays and special occasions. Rather than purchase gifts on her behalf, suggest homemade cards and small presents your child can buy with pocket money. Giving to others helps boost a child's self-esteem. Watch what happens when you say: "You're so thoughtful!" or "Thanks for helping!"

In Chapter 4, I talked about kids who smoke and use other drugs to shape their bodies. The pressure on kids to experiment with cigarettes, alcohol, and other substances is pervasive. One recent study of eighth-grade children showed that more than a third had tried marijuana while more than half had smoked tobacco. Whether at home or elsewhere, three out of four had tried alcohol. Apart from the obvious health risks linked with drug use, people who start smoking or drinking as children have a harder time quitting than those who start when they're older.

Decisions about alcohol and drug use are among the toughest a child will face. The choices she makes often determine who her friends are. But the opposite is also true: Her friends will likely influence the choices she makes. Many parents wait too long to discuss smoking and drinking with their kids. Kids need to know how to say "no" *before* they reach their teens.

How often have you or your friends told a small child that she'll put her eye out if she runs around with a sharp stick? (That one's in the Mother's Handbook.) You try to keep her safe by showing her how to cross the street or telling her what to do if a stranger should approach. Talking to your preteen about drugs and alcohol is equally important.

Kids need to know how to deal with offers of cigarettes, alcohol, and other drugs. One serious conversation isn't enough. Speak to your preteen about harmful substances whenever the topic comes up. There'll be plenty of news articles and television shows to cue you. Discuss ways to avoid being in situations where drugs are offered. And let your child know she has a right to say: "No thanks, I don't do that." There's nothing wrong with evasion. She can say she has to go home, and leave. Or say "Not right now." Take every opportunity to show your child she has the power to make the right choices. Kids who respect themselves are less likely to use tobacco or alcohol, or engage in other risky behaviors such as dieting, pill popping, and early sexual activity.

The Young Teen – Look Who's Talking

There's an old story about a child who never spoke. After years of anguish, his parents were amazed to hear him say: "This porridge is cold." "Why haven't you talked to us before?" they cried. His answer: "I've never had anything to complain about."

A young teen can easily become isolated from the family. Snug in her well-equipped private quarters, she feels self-contained. She may never have to help with the dishes or share a bathroom. One father I know was grateful that his daughter needed help with math—otherwise, he felt, she'd never speak to him! Kids who spend hours a day alone in their rooms don't learn how to function as members of the family, let alone the community. It's no wonder that kids get distorted images of reality when they spend most of their spare time sitting alone, watching TV, surfing the Net, or leafing through magazines.

Young teens tend to be especially self-conscious. Their need for acceptance is strong, and bonding with friends gives them the sense of belonging they crave. Still, no one can take the place of a caring parent. Keep talking to your teen, but most importantly, be a good listener. Show an honest curiosity about her day-to-day experiences. Resist the temptation to show shock or disgust, but feel free to express your opinions, briefly and honestly. Keep asking about *her* perceptions, letting her talk through the pros and cons of various situations. Be a mirror, rather than a judge, reflecting your teen's thoughts. Use phrases such as, "I think I hear you saying ..." and "That seems to make you feel ..." Of course, a good mirror doesn't always flatter, but it does let us see ourselves more clearly. Reassure your child that you're always on her side—whether she succeeds or fails. If she isn't afraid to bring home her report card, maybe she won't hesitate to bring home her boyfriend later on! Being approachable doesn't have to mean compromising your standards. If your child decides to experiment with cigarettes, you needn't permit smoking in your house. If she says, "*You drink—why shouldn't I?*" it's fair to point out that you're an adult.

Parents of teens often long for the time when their youngsters would sit and cuddle, or turn to them for a kiss "to make it better" after falling down. Your young teen still needs the power of touch—we all do! Studies show that hospital patients whose doctors give them a reassuring pat on the shoulder before surgery heal faster than patients whose doctors don't. A warm touch can promote physical, mental, and emotional health. Your teen may not let you hug her in front of her friends, but she probably won't flinch at a quick, private embrace. She might even accept a shoulder massage before she goes to sleep. It's important to keep "in touch" with kids—quite literally—no matter how grown-up they may seem.

The Older Teenager – The Juggler

An older teen often juggles a part-time job, hours of homework, extracurricular activities, relationships with friends, and the pressures of college applications and future career choices. It isn't the mad social whirl it appears to be. Too busy for family dinners, many a teen comes home to the microwave—and eats alone. A recent study of 7,000 teenagers found kids troubled more by loneliness than by anything else. Those interviewed wished they could spend more time with adults, especially their parents. When I went away on business trips during my daughters' high-school years, they said they missed me more than when they were little girls. Their need for support was related to the complexity of their lives.

Sports and fitness activities can offer kids a great outlet for releasing tension, but they can also be a *source* of stress. Kids often train so hard they reach a breaking point. They can take on so many activities they wear themselves out. If your child is good at several sports, she may be tempted to participate in too many. Other students and coaches may pressure her to join their teams. Help your child prioritize. And help her notice signs of stress such as irritability, headaches, extreme fatigue, loss of appetite, or a tendency to cry easily. Encourage her to take a break when she needs to recharge, and to explain her needs to her coach. She'll learn important lessons in accepting limits and speaking up.

Older teens are more likely to turn to drugs and alcohol if they haven't learned positive ways to cope with pressure. While a younger teen may drink or smoke to show off, an older teen may use alcohol or tobacco to relax or boost her confidence. It's not unusual to find teenagers "warming up" with a drink or two to feel more comfortable at a party. It's double jeopardy when a drinking teen's at the wheel of a car.

Should you let your teen drink at home? Perhaps there's no harm in offering a sip of wine on a special occasion, if the adults present demonstrate responsible drinking behavior. A child in high school may soon be away at college where she'll make her own choices. Practicing some adult behaviors while she's still under your roof may help. I don't think it's ever wise to offer a drink to other minors. For one thing, it's against the law. For another, it can have serious consequences.

Your older teen is developing a sense of identity along with values and beliefs of her own. She'll benefit from any healthy habit that gives her a sense of control in her daily life: relaxed breathing, moderate physical activity, talking over problems, writing in a journal. Parents, teachers, and adult friends play a critical role in putting kids at ease. The key is supporting young people to be themselves—not trying to sway them to fit *our* vision for their future. It's natural to have dreams for our children, and to try to provide opportunities we missed growing up, but our children have dreams of their own. The idea of a child's conforming—rather than spreading her wings—lies at the very root of weight and body-image problems.

Because You Asked about Stress and Relaxation

Q: Should I give my baby a pacifier? I see them everywhere, but I wonder if babies become too dependent on them. My nephew is two—and he won't give his up or go to bed without it.

A: *Pacifiers have their place, but I don't recommend giving one to a baby until nursing is well established, usually after four to six weeks. The more the baby sucks at the breast, the more milk you'll produce. Don't offer a pacifier to a baby who's slow to gain weight. It may be better for a baby who gains well and wants to suck often to have an orthodontic pacifier than to nurse each time she fusses, or to suck her fingers or thumbs. Give her the soother during the day, but not at bedtime—she'll be less likely to depend on it to get to sleep. Your nephew will eventually lose interest in his pacifier, but I wouldn't try to rush it. A cuddle at bedtime that includes a story and a lullaby may help him drop off to sleep without it.*

Q: My seven-month-old still wakes up every hour during the night to nurse. How can I get her to go longer between feedings? I'm exhausted from lack of sleep.

A: *Wakeful babies are a reality of life, but there are ways of helping them sleep for longer spells during the night. Some breastfed babies get in the habit of having too many "mini meals." To make sure she's hungry for her bedtime feeding, wait about two hours after her dinner of solid foods before nursing her again. When you do nurse, be sure to let her completely empty one breast before moving her to the other side (the last bit of milk from each breast has a higher concentration of fat, which will keep her satisfied longer). If she wakes up before two hours have passed, comfort her without feeding her unless she's howling. Over the next two to three weeks, gradually shift the time between night feedings from two hours to three hours, then four hours, and so on. Soon there'll only be one middle-of-the-night feeding, which your baby will eventually sleep right through. If you don't feel you're making any progress after a week or so, call a public health nurse, lactation consultant, or member of La Leche League for further advice and coaching.*

Q: I know it's not good for kids to watch too much TV, but my fourth grader and I enjoy a cuddle before bed while we watch our favorite sitcom. We find it a good way to relax at the end of the day, especially as we snack. What do you think?

A: *When my kids were that age, we often watched a TV program together at bedtime. I liked to watch TV with them so I knew what they were watching and could talk about it with them. Before we settled in front of the screen, snuggling together in an easy chair, we ate our snack in the kitchen. That way we didn't end up nibbling absent mindedly while viewing TV. Once in a while though, we broke with routine and shared a bowl of popcorn during TV time. When the girls spent an evening with a babysitter, I specified the programs and length of time they could watch. I didn't want them to go to bed with disturbing images in their minds. I'm not against television as long as it doesn't dominate family life, and kids watch age-appropriate programs.*

Q: My partner and I have full-time jobs and two young children. By the time we eat dinner, clean up, play with the kids, and get them to bed, we're exhausted. We just don't have time to be "easy."

A: *Let the kids help prepare dinner and clean up, so that you're working and talking together as a "team" from the moment you come home. Extend this idea to other household chores unless you can afford some outside help. But don't set the housekeeping standards too high. Is it more important to relax for a while each evening than to have a really tidy home? Is it okay to simplify meals on weeknights? Could you cut down on ironing with "easy care" clothing for everyone? Set aside some time to chat with the kids before they drift off to sleep. Make sure you and your partner have a little time alone together before you do the same. Small things can make your shared time more intimate. Face each other when you're talking—looking into each other's eyes—rather than sitting side-by-side in front of the tube.*

Q: Do you believe in setting a curfew for a teenager? My high-school son says no one else has one. He correctly points out that he's never given us a reason not to trust him.

A: *I think a teenager needs a curfew when he gets to the age where his parents no longer pick him up after an evening out. Let your son help you decide on a reasonable time for him to come home at night. My kids had a midnight curfew in the 10th grade, then got to stay up progressively later as they got older. They sometimes negotiated a later curfew for a special occasion. Teenagers need nine or 10 hours' sleep a night. Sometimes they need an excuse to leave a dicey situation and come home. Tell your son you love and trust him, but you want him to get his sleep without spending half the next day in bed—and tell him you always sleep easier once you know he's home.*

A Final Word ...

My mother often says, "I wouldn't want to be a parent in this day and age." Then my sister and I chime in: "But you *are* a parent in this day and age!" Of course, we know what she means. There are new challenges in bringing up today's kids. But parents of the new millennium can tap into the same lessons Nature provided when *our* parents were young. We just have to listen a little more closely—the world has become a noisier place!

Time hasn't changed a baby's amazing capacity to know when to eat and when to stop. She may be wearing designer booties, but she's still Nature's child! And today's parents are no less interested in responding to their children's needs. Many a modern mom and dad are surprised by the ferocity of their parental instincts.

We're all attracted to Nature's bounty. The diversity of plants and animals appeals to something deep within us. We just have to remind ourselves that people differ, too. Beauty comes in many sizes, shapes, and colors. Nature is forgiving. We work too hard and get a headache—it goes away. We get distracted and cut ourselves—the finger heals. Our adaptable bodies also enable us to correct mistakes and oversights related to eating, activity, and relaxation.

We can count on Nature to show us the way—and even to cut us a little slack. For our part, we have to pay attention. Nature speaks softly, and we're easily distracted. When we *do* pay attention, we see her generosity—an abundance of nourishing foods to fuel activities and maintain our bodies; an inborn ability to build strength through everyday activities; the capacity to renew ourselves through rest and relaxation.

It's *still* wonderful to be a parent "in this day and age!" Once, as I herded my little girls, an older friend said, "You're a lucky woman." She was right. When we count our blessings, the children who touch our lives are at the top of the list.

Selected References

Books

Berg, Frances M. *Afraid to Eat: Children and Teens in Weight Crisis.* Hettinger, ND: Healthy Weight Publishing Network, 1997.

Capaldi, Elizabeth D. *Why We Eat What We Eat: The Psychology of Eating.* Washington: American Psychological Association, 1996.

Coloroso, Barbara. *Kids Are Worth It!* Toronto: Somerville House Publishing, 1994.

Cook, Brian B., and Gordon W. Stewart. *Strength Basics: Your Guide to Resistance Training for Health and Optimal Performance.* Windsor, ON: Human Kinetics, 1996.

Davies, Máire Messenger. *Fake, Fact, and Fantasy: Children's Interpretations of Television Reality.* Mahwah, NJ: Lawrence Erlbaum Associates, 1997.

Harris, Judith Rich. *The Nurture Assumption: Why Children Turn Out the Way They Do.* New York: The Free Press, Simon & Schuster Inc., 1998.

Joneja, Janice V. *Dietary Management of Food Allergies and Intolerances: A Comprehensive Guide.* Vancouver: J.A. Hall Publications Ltd., 1997.

McNicol, Jane. *The Great Big Food Experiment: How to Identify—and Control—Your Child's Food Intolerances.* Toronto: Stoddart, 1990.

Mahan, Kathleen L., and Sylvia Escott-Stump. *Krause's Food, Nutrition, & Diet Therapy.* Philadelphia: W. B. Saunders Company, 2000.

Maté, Gabor. *Scattered Minds: A New Look at the Origins and Healing of Attention Deficit Disorder.* Toronto: Alfred A. Knopf, 1999.

Melina, Vesanto, et al. *Becoming Vegetarian: The Complete Guide to Adopting a Healthy Vegetarian Diet.* Toronto: Macmillan Canada, 1994.

Pipher, Mary. *Reviving Ophelia: Saving the Selves of Adolescent Girls.* New York: Ballantine Books, 1994.

Roberts, Susan B., and Melvin B. Heyman. *Feeding Your Child for Lifelong Health.* New York and Toronto: Bantam Books, 1999.

Satter, Ellyn. *How to Get Your Child to Eat ... But Not Too Much.* Palo Alto: Bull Publishing, 1987.

Satter, Ellyn. *Secrets of Feeding a Healthy Family.* Madison, WI: Kelcy Press, 1999.

Stewart, Gordon W. *Active Living: The Miracle Medicine for a Long and Healthy Life.* Windsor, ON: Human Kinetics, 1995.

Toews, Judy, and Nicole Parton. *Never Say Diet!* Toronto: Key Porter Books, 1998.

Journal Articles

Anon. "Survey Results Link Parental Physical Activity to Children's Behaviors." *WIN Notes* (National Institutes of Health) 4 (2): 2, 1998.

Berg, F. M. "Breaking Free: The Health at Any Size Revolution." *Healthy Weight Journal* 14: 15, 2000.

Birch, L. L. "Children's Food Acceptance Patterns." *Nutrition Today* 31 (6): 234, 1996.

Epstein, L. H., et al. "Treatment of Pediatric Obesity." *Pediatrics* 101: 554, 1998.

Field, A. E., et al. "Exposure to the Mass Media and Weight Concerns Among Girls." *Pediatrics* 103 (3): 36, 1999.

Hill, J. O. "Genetic and Environmental Contributions To Obesity." *American J. Clinical Nutrition* 68: 991, 1998.

Kohl, H. W. and K. E. Hobbs. "Development of Physical Activity Behaviors Among Children and Adolescents." *Pediatrics Supplement* 101: 549, 1998.

Kotz, K., and M. Story. "Food Advertisements During Children's Saturday Morning Television Programming: Are They Consistent with Dietary Recommendations?" *J. American Dietetic Assoc.* 94 (11): 1,296, 1994.

Neumark-Sztainer, D., et al. "Beliefs and Attitudes about Obesity among Teachers and School Health Care Providers Working with Adolescents." *J. Nutrition Education* 31: 3, 1999.

Story, M., and J. E. "Do Young Children Instinctively Know What to Eat? The Studies of Clara Davis Revisited." *New England Journal of Medicine* 316 (2): 103, 1987.

Reports

Canadian Paediatric Society, Dietitians of Canada, Health Canada. *Statement of the Joint Working Group: Nutrition for Healthy Term Infants*. Minister of Public Works and Government Services Canada, 1998.

Health Canada. *Canada's Food Guide to Healthy Eating: Focus on Preschoolers*. Ottawa: Minister of Supplies and Services Canada, 1995.

Health Canada. *Nutrition for a Healthy Pregnancy: National Guidelines for the Childbearing Years*. Ottawa: Minister of Public Works and Government Services Canada, 1999.

Kochan-Vintinner, Angela. *Active Living During Pregnancy: Physical Activity Guidelines for Mother and Baby*. Ottawa: Canadian Society for Exercise Physiology, 1999.

McCreary Centre Society. *Healthy Connections: Listening to BC Youth*. Burnaby, B.C., 1999.

Acknowledgments

I'm indebted to child-feeding expert Ellyn Satter of Wisconsin, whose "golden rule" of shared responsibility between parents and children has provided the foundation for my advice to parents for many years. Colorado parenting educator Barbara Coloroso has also inspired me, as has author, editor, and size-acceptance advocate Frances Berg of North Dakota. I'm grateful to all of the parents who have shared their nutrition concerns with me. We've learned a great deal working together.

My home province of British Columbia has a terrific network of community nutritionists and public health nurses. I'm especially grateful to nutritionists Cathy Richards and Helen Lutz, who reviewed parts of the manuscript and offered suggestions.

I also owe a debt of thanks to B.C.'s Gordon Stewart—author, columnist, and health and fitness consultant—for teaching me about active living and kindly reviewing the chapter on activity. And I thank my colleague Judith Banfield, child development specialist and lactation consultant, for her insights and helpful suggestions. Thanks to B.C. occupational therapists Murielle Perrin and Laura Ford, and elementary school counselor Barbara Martin for their helpful tips.

I could never have written this book without the backing of my wonderful family, including my parents Gordon and Jeanne McAfee and my sister Jennifer Angell. Thanks to my daughters Sarah and Erica, who showed me that Nature's lessons really work. And an extra hug for my husband David, who cooked most of our meals while I was busy writing about the subject!

Nicole Parton has been indispensable as an editor, researcher, and supporter. As always, Nicole and I are grateful to Graham Harrop for his giant talent and warm friendship. Our very special thanks to Clare McKeon at Key Porter Books, for encouragement and advice, and her marvelous sense of fun, and to our wonderful editor Linda Pruessen.

Index

digestive problems, 114, 117-8
effect on behavior, 129, 131
effect on sleeping through the
night, 95, 186
encouraging healthy choices,
31-32, 34, 39-40, 45, 46, 59-61,
86-88, 100-4, 106-7, 110-6
environment for healthy, 31,
39-40, 87-88, 94, 96-98, 104,
107, 108, 124
guidelines for balanced eating,
116, 124, 128, 134, 142-4
importance of variety to health,
13, 20, 26, 28, 112-6
judging baby's needs, 106-7
judging quantities, 23-26, 33,
106-7, 136
picky and finicky eaters, 13, 17,
29-30, 39, 60, 100-1, 106, 126
principle of shared responsibility,
14, 21-22, 24, 32-35, 60, 87
rejection of, 23-24, 28-31, 38,
94-95, 98
restrained eating, 71, 73-75
restaurants, 45, 64, 97, 113
role of schools, 56, 61
serving sizes, 33-34, 64
signs of an eating disorder, 78-79
social aspects, 20-21, 30-31, 33-34,
45, 61, 83, 88, 96-97, 107, 109
strategies to lessen conflict,
33-34, 45, 61, 104, 172
introducing solid foods, 28, 94-95,
121-3, (vegetarian) 138-9
related to television, 47-50, 58,
60-61, 88, 100
super-tasters, 29
unhurried, 87-8, 94, 96, 102
vegetarian, 30, 75, 105-6, 112,
138-9

See also appetite, body wisdom,
diets, dieting, eating disorders,
food, junk food, salt, snacking,
sugar, teeth
eating disorders, 12, 15, 20-21, 42,
63, 64, 73-79
anorexia nervosa, 51, 76-77
binge eating disorder, 74-5, 77-78
bulimia nervosa, 76-77
compulsive exercising, 76-78,
84, 160-1
disguised, 75
family counseling, 79, 84
reverse anorexia, 78
role of schools, 56-57
signs of, 78-79
exercise, 145-65
active living defined, 146-7
benefits of, 146-9
breastfeeding, 149-50
college life, 165
compulsive, 76-78, 84, 160-1
encouraging healthy choices,
45, 62, 64, 83, 101-2, 164
endorphins, 146
in reverse anorexia, 78
inactivity and daily life, 15,
47-49, 62, 64, 83, 145, 157,
159, 164
infants, 151
infant walker hazard, 152-3
lactic acid buildup, 150
negative effect of
regimentation, 71
older babies, 151-3
primary schoolers, 163-4
related to sleep, 171
role of schools, 56-57, 131, 156-8
sexual activity, 148-9, 158
sports nutrition, 134-6